DID YOU KNOW?

- Hypertension is the third leading cause of death in this country.
- The higher your blood pressure, the shorter your life expectancy.
- Hypertension strikes one out of three African-Americans, as compared to one out of four Caucasians.
- Up until the age of sixty, women are less likely than men to develop high blood pressure, but after age sixty women take the lead.
- Vegetarians have lower blood pressure levels than nonvegetarians and they tend to develop hypertension less often.
- Approximately 60 percent of hypertensive Americans are overweight—but in many cases, losing just ten or twenty pounds can bring blood pressure down to normal levels.
- Obesity in early adulthood, between the ages of twenty and thirty, significantly increases the risk of developing hypertension later on.
- Aspirin, ibuprofen, oral contraceptives, decongestants, corticosteroids—and a host of other over-the-counter and prescription drugs—can elevate your blood pressure.

LEARN WHAT YOU NEED TO KNOW ABOUT THIS DISEASE IN...
WHAT YOUR DOCTOR MAY NOT TELL YOU ABOUT™ HYPERTENSION

"A groundbreaking program. Everyone who wants to prevent—or even reverse—hypertension should read this book."
—**Allen Montgomery, R.Ph., CEO & president, American Nutraceutical Association**

more...

"Absolutely essential reading....Dr. Houston's extraordinary understanding of dietary factors underlying hypertension is apparent throughout the book. It provides a clear-cut and do-able plan for lowering blood pressure using the best of alternative and traditional medicine."
—**Loren Cordain, Ph.D., author of** *The Paleo Diet*

"Truly masterful....This is a book that can help save lives. It represents the best that personalized preventive medicine has to offer....A must read."
—**Jeffrey Bland, Ph.D., FACN, CNS, chairman, Institute for Functional Medicine**

"This is the most comprehensive and up-to-date book on hypertension and nutrition I have ever read....Written by the most authoritative figure in the field. Buy one for yourself, and one for your doctor."
—**Robert Crayhon, M.S., author of** *Robert Crayhon's Nutrition Made Simple*

"Dr. Houston offers easy-to-understand data on traditional, complementary, and alternative therapies, exposing readers to a wide range of management options for hypertension."
—**Catherine Ulbricht, PharmD., R.Ph., founder, Natural Standard, and editor,** *Journal of Herbal Pharmacotherapy*

"Dr. Houston offers a simple, easy-to-understand guide....This book is a must for laypersons and clinicians....A must for every bookshelf."
—**Bernd Wollschlaeger, M.D., F.A.A.F.P., clinical assistant professor of medicine and family medicine, University of Miami School of Medicine**

WHAT YOUR DOCTOR MAY *NOT* TELL YOU ABOUT™
HYPERTENSION

The Revolutionary Nutrition and Lifestyle Program to Help Fight High Blood Pressure

---

MARK HOUSTON, M.D.
with BARRY FOX, Ph.D.,
and NADINE TAYLOR, M.S., R.D.

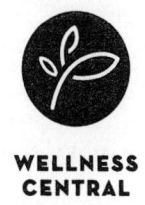

WELLNESS CENTRAL

NEW YORK   BOSTON

The information herein is not intended to replace the services of trained health professionals, or be a substitute for medical advice. You are advised to consult with your health care professional with regard to matters relating to your health, and in particular regarding matters that may require diagnosis or medical attention.

Copyright © 2003 by Mark Houston, M.D., Barry Fox, Ph.D., and Nadine Taylor, M.S., R.D.
All rights reserved. Except as permitted under the U.S. Copyright Act of 1976, no part of this publication may be reproduced, distributed, or transmitted in any form or by any means, or stored in a database or retrieval system, without the prior written permission of the publisher.

The title of the series What Your Doctor May Not Tell You About . . . and the related trade dress are trademarks owned by Grand Central Publishing and may not be used without permission.

Wellness Central
Hachette Book Group
237 Park Avenue
New York, NY 10017

Visit our Web site at www.HachetteBookGroup.com.

Wellness Central is an imprint of Grand Central Publishing.
The Wellness Central name and logo is a trademark of Hachette Book Group, Inc.

Printed in the United States of America

First Edition: October 2003
10 9 8 7 6 5

Library of Congress Cataloging-in-Publication Data
Houston, Mark
    What your doctor may not tell you about hypertension : the revolutionary nutrition and lifestyle program to help fight high blood pressure / Mark Houston, with Barry Fox and Nadine Taylor.
        p. cm.
    Includes bibliographical references and index.
    ISBN 978-0-446-69084-3
    1. Hypertension—Popular works. 2. Hypertension—Alternative treatment. I. Fox, Barry. II. Taylor, Nadine. III. Title

RC685.H8H654 2003
616.1'32—dc21   2003043269

Book design by Charles A. Sutherland
Cover design by Diane Luger

Acknowledgments

I acknowledge and dedicate this book to my parents, R.R. and Mary Ruth Houston, and Laurie Hays, my wife, for their continued support.

I would also like to thank Monica Coote, C.N., for preparing the recipes for this book.

Contents

Introduction	ix
CHAPTER 1. The Symptomless Disease	1
CHAPTER 2. What Sends Your Blood Pressure Soaring?	14
CHAPTER 3. The Multifaceted Solution	45
CHAPTER 4. The *Hypertension Institute Program*	89
CHAPTER 5. The DASH Diet	100
CHAPTER 6. Design Your Own Diet	131
CHAPTER 7. Prime the Pump with Exercise	155
CHAPTER 8. De-Stress Your Life	177
CHAPTER 9. If Medicine Is Necessary	186
CHAPTER 10. The Future Is Yours	219
Appendix. A Closer Look at the Studies	224
Notes	253
Index	279

Introduction

Over 50 million Americans suffer from hypertension, the "silent killer" that greatly increases your risk of suffering a heart attack, congestive heart failure, or stroke, or developing kidney failure, vision loss, or other problems.

Physicians are, quite rightly, concerned about hypertension. They monitor it carefully and often treat it aggressively, lest it slip out of control and quietly wreak havoc on your body. If your blood pressure is high, your doctor will check it regularly, and most likely prescribe one or more of the numerous antihypertensive medications. Your physician will also suggest that you drop down to your ideal weight if you're carrying too many pounds, exercise regularly, eat a healthful diet, and make other health and lifestyle changes.

In theory, this approach should be fairly successful—and it is, for many people. Unfortunately, due in large part to the side effects and cost of the drugs, this approach is not nearly as successful as we'd like it to be. Almost one third of those with hypertension don't even realize they have it, and well over half of those who know they have it are not being treated adequately. Of the more than 50 million hypertensive Americans, fewer than 14 million have it under control.

We need to broaden our approach to treating elevated blood pressure and find new, easy-to-tolerate, inexpensive treatments that people can easily incorporate into their lives. Fortunately, there are such treatments, although most physicians either don't know about them or won't pass the information on to their patients. Either way, the odds are your doctor won't tell you about the voluminous research showing, for example, that magnesium, potassium, calcium, vitamin C, omega-3 fatty acids, olive oil, coenzyme Q_{10}, and other common nutrients, foods, and supplements may lower your systolic blood pressure by 10 mm Hg or more! Neither will he or she explain that olive oil, vitamin C, and other substances may reduce your diastolic pressure 5 mm Hg or more! These are impressive reductions, the kind that physicians would love to see when treating patients with standard medicines. And these reductions in blood pressure come without the strong side effects or high cost that typically accompanies medication use.

Please don't misunderstand. The medicines used to control blood pressure are very helpful; they've saved countless lives. But, like everything else in life, they have their limits. That's why doctors should be telling their patients about other, nonmedicinal approaches. And that's why we wrote this book.

In the chapters that follow, you'll learn all about hypertension: what it is and how it harms us. Then you'll delve into the exciting new world of nutraceuticals, those foods and supplements that have medicinal properties. You'll learn how diet in general, and various foods and supplements in particular, can help you keep your blood pressure under control. You'll also learn how to use exercise, stress reduction, and other lifestyle habits to aid in this process. All the information in this book is backed by solid science.

If you were to ask the average physician about nutrients and hypertension, he or she would undoubtedly tell you to eat less salt, lose weight, exercise, and get plenty of calcium and potassium. That's good advice, but it's only the beginning. It's time to move into the twenty-first century with a new, improved, more thorough approach to conquering hypertension, at long last.

WHAT YOUR DOCTOR MAY *NOT* TELL YOU ABOUT™
HYPERTENSION

Chapter 1

The Symptomless Disease

A woman lies dead in her hospital bed. The only sound in the room is the ominous whine of a heart monitor, which proclaims to one and all that her heart has, at last, ceased functioning.

A fifty-six-year-old man walks briskly down a busy avenue on his way to work. Suddenly his face contorts with pain. He drops his briefcase, clutches his head in agony, and is dead before he hits the ground.

An elderly woman lies in a hospital bed, undergoing kidney dialysis. These thrice-weekly treatments leave her exhausted, but without them she would die.

A businessman and father of three sits in an easy chair and sighs as he gazes out the window. He has given up the golfing he loved so much because, with his heart failing, he just hasn't got the energy to play anymore. That's true even if he spends 95 percent of his time in a golf cart.

Although each of these people suffered from a distinctly different disease, in the end they all died of the same underlying problem—*hypertension*, commonly called high blood pressure. Hypertension is often called the silent killer because it usually exhibits no obvious symptoms until the blood pressure is very high. Its victims don't feel anything out of the ordinary and have no idea that something is amiss until plenty of damage has been done. But make no mistake: Hypertension is a killer. If you have uncontrolled high blood pressure, you also have an increased risk of stroke, heart attack, heart failure, and kidney failure. And with each slight rise in your blood pressure, the risk increases. Depending on how high your pressure goes, you may be as much as seven to ten times more likely to have a stroke; three times more likely to develop coronary heart disease (blocked heart vessels); and six times more likely to develop congestive heart failure than those with normal blood pressure.[1]

It's the utter lack of pain or any other warning signs that makes mild to moderate hypertension so insidious. You would know it if your leg was broken; you couldn't miss the pain, and you'd rush to the doctor to get it X-rayed and splinted. Similarly, if the valve separating your food pipe from your stomach wasn't doing its job, you'd feel the unmistakable sting of heartburn and you'd start rummaging through your medicine cabinet for antacids. And if your bronchial tubes went into spasm, bringing on an asthma attack, you'd be sure to grab your inhaler. But since you can't feel, hear, taste, or see the signs of hypertension, you can easily ignore it.

Far from a rare occurrence (it's third on the most deadly disease list, right behind heart disease and cancer), hypertension strikes one out of every four adult Americans—over 50 million people. It's the disease that doctors see more often than any other and the one that prompts them to write the most prescriptions. Yet it continues to devastate: In 1999 alone, hypertension killed nearly 43,000 Americans and was a major contributing factor to 227,000 other deaths.

But because it's usually symptomless, hypertension is also one of our most under-treated ailments. Almost one third of those with hypertension (15 million Americans) don't even know they have it and are, therefore, doing nothing to prevent or treat it. Even worse, of the 35 million Americans who *do* know they have the disease, 13.1 million are being inadequately treated, and another 7.4 million are receiving no treatment at all. That's a staggering number of walking time bombs! The bottom line is only 13.7 million of the 50 million Americans with hypertension—a mere 27.4 percent—are both aware they've got the disease *and* controlling it.

HOW DOES EXCESS PRESSURE HARM US?

Why does it matter if blood pressure rises? After all, the amount of blood doesn't change, the red blood cells keep delivering oxygen, and the white blood cells still maintain their protective vigil. A blood sample taken from someone with hypertension wouldn't look different under the microscope from one taken from a healthy person.

The problem is too much pressure in the cardiovascular system, which consists of the *heart* and the *blood vessels* (*arteries*, *veins*, and *capillaries*). The arteries carry blood away from the heart, the veins carry it to the heart, and the capillaries are the tiny blood vessels that actually deliver the blood to the tissues. With hypertension, we're primarily concerned with the arteries, as they bear the brunt of the pressure exerted by each heartbeat. Because of this, the arteries have thicker, elastic, and muscular walls that relax and open wide as the blood courses through them. Veins, on the other hand, have much thinner walls and are not as prone to damage from hypertension because they're not subjected to nearly as much force.

Too much pressure within the cardiovascular system can hurt you in several ways. The excess force generated by the coursing of the blood against blood vessel walls can damage their all-important lining (the *endothelium*). This is more dangerous than it sounds because the cells that make up the endothelium secrete hormones and substances that help control the blood pressure, stickiness of the blood, growth of the blood vessel wall, and other factors vitally important to cardiovascular health. Damage to the endothelium speeds up what's called hardening of the arteries (*atherosclerosis*), a process that affects all of us as we age. These stiffened, narrowed arteries have a hard time supplying the body with enough oxygen and nutrients, which means the tissues and organs that they serve can be damaged. For example, if the arteries in your eye are afflicted, your vision may suffer. If the arteries in your kidneys are damaged, you may develop kidney disease or kidney failure and wind up on dialysis. If the arteries supplying your heart muscle are damaged, you can develop blockages that can cause a heart attack. And if the arteries in your brain are affected, you may form blockages that can trigger a stroke. (See Chapter 2 for a more thorough explanation of the effects of hypertension on the body.)

HOW DO I KNOW IF MY BLOOD PRESSURE IS TOO HIGH?

Since you usually don't feel pain or any other symptoms, you probably won't know you've got a problem. That's why regular medical examinations, complete with blood pressure checks, are vital.

Your physician or nurse will usually read your blood pressure with a *sphygmomanometer*, that familiar cuff connected to a measuring device that looks something like a big thermometer. The cuff is wrapped snugly around your upper arm and inflated until it stops the blood flow in one of your arm's major arteries (the *brachial artery*). Then the cuff is slowly deflated while your physician or nurse listens with a stethoscope for the faint but clear tapping sound that indicates the blood is coursing through the artery once more. When this sound begins, the physician notes the reading on the sphygmomanometer, which is measured in millimeters of mercury (mm Hg). This first reading is the *systolic blood pressure* (*SBP*), the pressure exerted by the blood on the artery walls each time your heart beats.

The sounds change as the cuff continues to deflate, and when they are no longer heard, another measurement is noted. This is the *diastolic blood pressure* (*DBP*), the pressure exerted by the blood on the walls of your arteries when your heart is at rest between beats. The overall reading is expressed as a fraction, with the systolic on top and the diastolic underneath, as in 120/80. *Hypertension* is a condition in which the blood pressure exceeds normal limits most or all of the time. A reading of less than 120/80 mm Hg is considered normal, 120–130/80–90 is prehypertensive, a systolic pressure of 140 mm Hg or higher and/or a diastolic pressure of 90 mm Hg or higher is considered hypertensive.

Essential hypertension is high blood pressure that has no definite or known cause, which is the case 90 to 95 percent of the time. Although the cause is unknown, there is clearly a genetic component, as it tends to run in families. *Secondary hypertension* is high blood pressure due to another condition such as kidney disease, tumors, diseases of the endocrine system, blockages in the arteries of the kidneys, obesity, coarctation (narrowing) of the aorta, a variety of uncommon or rare disorders, and the use of certain prescription or nonprescription medications.

> ### SOUNDING OUT YOUR BLOOD PRESSURE
>
> There's more to reading blood pressure than listening for the first and last sounds; it's not just "sound on, sound off." As the physician releases the pressure on the cuff wrapped around the arm, the sound evolves through five phases, which are known as Korotkoff sounds.
>
> - Phase I—The doctor hears faint but clear tapping sounds, which gradually become more intense.
> - Phase II—The doctor begins to hear a swishing sound, or murmur.
> - Phase III—The sound becomes crisper, more intense.
> - Phase IV—The sound becomes muffled and soft; there's a blowing quality to the sound.
> - Phase V—The sound vanishes.

WHAT'S NORMAL AND WHAT'S NOT?

Here's the official word on blood pressure readings for those age eighteen and older, straight from the Seventh Report of the Joint National Committee on Prevention, Detection, Evaluation, and Treatment of High Blood Pressure,[2] a prestigious group of experts gathered together to set standards for the treatment of hypertension.

- Normal blood pressure—Systolic pressure less than 120 and diastolic pressure less than 80.
- Prehypertension—Systolic pressure 120–139 or diastolic pressure 80–89.

If *either* the systolic blood pressure is above 139 or the diastolic pressure tops 89, you have hypertension. There are two stages of hypertension:

- Stage 1 hypertension—Systolic pressure 140–159 *or* diastolic pressure 90–99.
- Stage 2 hypertension—Systolic pressure greater than or equal to 160 *or* diastolic pressure greater than or equal to 100.

Although they don't agree exactly where the lines between one category and the next should fall, the major health organizations agree on the seriousness of the problem. The American Heart Association, for example, has three classifications: blood pressure of less than 120/80 is normal for adults; a reading of 120–139/80–89 signals prehypertension and requires careful watching; elevated hypertension is a reading of 140/90 or above.

But don't breathe a sigh of relief and decide that you don't have much to worry about if you have, say, stage 1 hypertension. The latest studies indicate that even those who fall into the stage 1 category have a 31 percent greater risk of heart attack, almost twice the risk of stroke, and a 43 percent increase in death rate, compared to those in the normal to high-normal category. In fact, 60 percent of the disease, disability, and fatalities caused by hypertension occurs among those with stage 1 of the disease, and 32 percent of the deaths due to hypertension-related heart disease occurs in those with a systolic blood pressure of *less than 140 mm Hg.*

WHY CAN'T WE SOLVE THE PROBLEM?

With over 50 million victims in this country alone, hypertension is clearly a major health problem. It's no wonder, then, that pharmaceutical companies have spent billions of dollars developing numerous drugs to decrease elevated blood pressure, and that the federal government funds many research studies investigating new approaches. Yet less than one third of those with hypertension have it under control. Awareness of the problem is one factor, but a staggering number of people who know they have high blood pressure either don't take their medications properly or simply do nothing at all. In fact, about 50 percent of hypertensives never even fill their prescriptions.

A large part of the problem is the high cost of hypertension drugs and their potential side effects, which include fatigue, depression, sexual dysfunction, sedation, dry mouth, cough, dizziness, headache, nausea, diarrhea, constipation, rash, itching, flushing, and swelling of the ankle or leg. But whatever the reason, tens of millions of people are walking around with uncontrolled hypertension, as the silent killer weakens their arteries, taxes their hearts, corrodes arteries in their brains, threatens their eyesight, and eats away at their kidneys. But all of this is unnecessary, because the hypertension medications actually do a very good job of controlling the disease.

THE SAFE, NATURAL, AND EFFECTIVE ALTERNATIVE

Yet as good as the medications are, they really aren't the best answer to the hypertension problem. We need a new approach, something safe, natural, effective, comprehensive, and yet easy to tolerate. Something that not only lowers blood pressure, but also improves the health of the arteries, without side effects. And something people can stick with forever. That something is the *Hypertension Institute Program* that I developed at the

Hypertension Institute, where I've treated thousands of patients with high blood pressure over the past thirteen years.

Not too long ago, I was like any other hypertension and internal medicine specialist, routinely prescribing the latest medicines for my hypertensive patients. I was doing everything right: I was (and continue to be) an Associate Clinical Professor of Medicine at the Vanderbilt University School of Medicine, and Director of the Hypertension Institute in Nashville, Tennessee, where I practice at Saint Thomas Medical Group and Saint Thomas Hospital. I personally conducted over seventy-five research studies on hypertension, published over 120 medical articles, and wrote two handbooks that health care providers use as guides for treating hypertension and understanding vascular biology. I also served as a consulting reviewer for the editorial board for numerous peer-reviewed medical journals such as the *Journal of the American Medical Association*, the *New England Journal of Medicine*, the *Archives of Internal Medicine*, the *American Journal of Hypertension*, and *Human Hypertension*.

Despite my firm footing in standard medicine, I began looking into the alternative literature because I wanted to design a healthy-heart, healthy-blood-vessel, and age-management program for myself—something that included nutrition, dietary supplements, and *nutraceuticals* (components of foods or dietary supplements that have medicinal or therapeutic uses). But since I knew that traditional medicine didn't adequately address these issues, I turned to complementary and integrative medicine, figuring I might be able to pick up a few tips there. As I began to read more and more, I was astonished to find a wealth of convincing basic science and clinical studies showing that certain vitamins, minerals, nutraceuticals, dietary supplements, and other food-related substances could do exactly what I wanted. I was especially impressed with the research on hypertension. According to these scientific studies, many foods, antioxidants, flavonoids, fatty acids, vitamins, minerals, macro- and micronutrients can lower blood pressure relatively quickly and safely—without side effects. For example, vitamin C can lower systolic blood pressure by 11 mm Hg, and coenzyme Q_{10} can lower it an amazing 14 mm Hg!

Once I'd read the research describing the beneficial effects of these foods and other substances on high blood pressure, I started giving my new patients a choice of treatments. I'd say, "Would you like me to treat your high blood pressure with standard medicine? Or would you rather try more natural treatments, like vitamins, minerals, or other supplements, plus diet and exercise? Or, as a third option, what about a mix of the two approaches?" Every one of them chose the mixed standard and natural approach, then later on wanted to move to an all-natural approach if and when it was safe and appropriate.

Over a period of several years, I've come up with a list of nutraceuticals that can significantly and safely lower high blood pressure without the side effects common to medications. I've combined these substances to make up what I call the VasoGuard Therapy, an all-natural, scientifically valid recipe for lowering hypertension. You can buy the ingredients (individually or in combination) at various supermarkets, pharmacies, health food, or vitamin stores.[3] (We'll discuss the VasoGuard Therapy in Chapter 4.)

But supplements are only a part of the answer, because every good program for reducing hypertension must also include the DASH-I and DASH-II diets. (DASH stands for Dietary Approaches to Stop Hypertension.) The DASH-I diet emphasizes fruits, vegetables, and low-fat dairy products. It's also low in saturated fat, cholesterol, and total fat. The DASH-II diet includes all of these elements but adds sodium restriction. Both have been proven to reduce blood pressure significantly, particularly DASH-II, and both are endorsed by the American Heart Association, the Joint National Committee on Prevention, Detection, Evaluation, and Treatment of High Blood Pressure, and the World Health Organization, plus the International, European, and American Societies of Hypertension. (The DASH diets are thoroughly explained in Chapter 5.)

My VasoGuard Therapy plus the modified DASH diet are the beginnings of my *Hypertension Institute Program*. To these I add other dietary measures, exercise, weight loss, stress reduction, cutting back on alcohol and caffeine, giving up tobacco, plus the judicious use of medicines as needed. Together these elements make up what I believe is the safest, most effective program for controlling hypertension in existence today.

THE SCIENCE BEHIND THE PROGRAM

As a physician and scientist, I've conducted numerous, rigorous studies on hypertension and published over 120 articles on the topic in peer-reviewed medical journals. I'm definitely not one who rushes to endorse half-baked ideas or introduce any new approach until it's supported by a very thick stack of scientific literature—plus a great deal of hands-on, real-life experience. But I have no worries about the scientific validity of using nutrition, some dietary supplements, vitamins, minerals, and nutraceuticals as "medicine" for hypertension. The medical literature is positively overflowing with studies—over 1,000 of them—that demonstrate the value of various natural substances and foods in lowering elevated blood pressure. A sampling of some of the most important studies can be found in Chapter 3.

But it's not just the nutraceuticals in my VasoGuard Therapy that have been subjected to rigorous scientific tests. The DASH diets and other parts of my *Hypertension Institute Program* have also been thoroughly studied. Without reservation, I can assure you that this program is based on real science: It's not just a compilation of far-fetched ideas.

THE FULL HYPERTENSION INSTITUTE PROGRAM

Although some people may be tempted to take the VasoGuard supplements alone and forget about the rest of the program, I must emphasize that there are no magic pills or instant cures for high blood pressure. Controlling hypertension is a lifelong battle that involves a full commitment to all of the elements that will be addressed in this book: the modified DASH diet, exercise, maintaining your ideal weight, reasonably restricting alcohol and caffeine, stopping smoking, and the other parts of the *Hypertension Institute Program*. But once you make that commitment, your blood pressure can drop significantly and your health can improve immeasurably.

Here's the ten-point program in a nutshell:

1. See your physician regularly.
2. Adopt the specially modified DASH diet.
3. Use the VasoGuard Therapy.
4. Exercise regularly.
5. Maintain your ideal weight.
6. De-stress your life.
7. Reduce your alcohol intake to a reasonable level.
8. Cut back on the caffeine.

9. Say goodbye to smoking and tobacco products.
10. Use standard medicines as necessary.

Now that you've been introduced to the basics of the *Hypertension Institute Program*, let's take a closer look at what may be driving your blood pressure up in the first place.

Chapter 2

What Sends Your Blood Pressure Soaring?

Sixty, seventy, perhaps eighty times a minute, your heart contracts and pumps freshly oxygenated blood through the aorta, the giant artery rising up and away from your heart. Some of that blood flows out into a network of progressively smaller arteries that snake their way through your chest, arms, neck, and head. Another portion of the blood finds its way to your liver, kidneys, and other mid-body areas, while the rest travels through the aorta until the artery forks, with either branch continuing down through your lower body and into each corresponding leg.

No matter what its destination, the blood follows a similar path: from the aorta, through larger then progressively smaller arteries, then finally into the tiny capillaries where oxygen and nutrients are exchanged for waste products at the cellular level. Having performed these duties, the blood begins its journey back to the heart through a series of ever larger veins. The entire process is dependent upon the ceaseless beating of the heart, plus a fairly constant amount of pressure in the system.

A LOOK AT THE PLUMBING

When we talk about elevated blood pressure, the first thing we think of is the heart. After all, there's a lot going on in the heart. It beats sixty to ninety times per minute, or about 100,000 times a day. During an average lifetime, it will beat more than 2.5 billion times, pumping about 1 million barrels worth of blood throughout your body. But there's a lot going on in the blood vessels, too. They automatically deliver greater or lesser amounts of blood to the tissues exactly when it's needed.

Together, the heart and the blood vessels make up the *cardiovascular system*, a complex but highly efficient system that delivers oxygen and nutrients to every cell in the body, exchanging them for waste products that are swept away for disposal or recycling.

The heart is essentially four empty chambers surrounded by muscle. Used blood from all over the body enters into the top right chamber (right atrium), rests there for just a moment, then drops down into the bottom right chamber (right ventricle). When the heart beats (when the muscle surrounding the heart squeezes), the used blood in the bottom right chamber shoots out of the heart and through an artery into the lungs. There, the blood releases the load of carbon dioxide it's been carrying, picks up a fresh load of oxygen, and returns to the heart.

Now entering the heart for the second time, the oxygen-rich blood goes into the top left chamber (left atrium). It rests there for just a moment before dropping into the bottom left chamber (left ventricle). The bottom left chamber is the real workhorse of the heart, as it has to propel fresh blood completely out of the heart and through an incredibly long series of arteries that tunnel throughout the body into every limb and organ.

We normally think of the arteries and veins as being like the plumbing pipes in our houses, just lying there passively while things pass through them. But the vascular system is more than just a bunch of pipes. It functions as an organ, just like the heart, with a series of tasks it must perform in order to keep the blood flowing smoothly. And like all living tissue, it can be damaged, which causes certain important body functions to go awry.

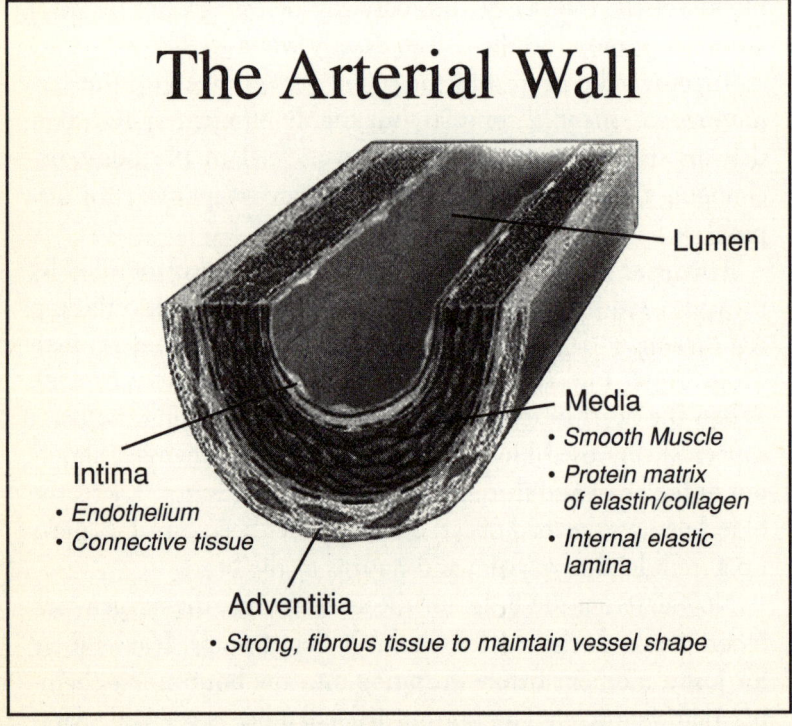

Fig. 2.1

Although the vascular system is made up of both arteries and veins, it's the arteries that are the real problem in hypertension. Look at the diagram of the artery on the previous page. It's not just one substance like a hose—a certain thickness of "artery stuff." Instead, it's made up of several layers of different substances, each with different capabilities, different tasks, and different vulnerabilities. In hypertension, we're primarily concerned with the innermost wall of the artery, the lining—called the *endothelium*—and with the muscular media.

The endothelium is, in fact, an endocrine organ,[1] which means that it manufactures and secretes hormones locally and directly into the bloodstream. These hormones deliver messages, instructing arteries, blood, body tissues, and other organs to do, or not to do, various things. And the endothelium is a pretty big organ; in fact, it's the largest in the body, weighing in at nearly five pounds. If you were to peel it out of the arteries and lay it flat, it would take up about 14,000 square feet in surface area—that's the size of six and one half tennis courts!

Besides releasing numerous hormones and other substances, the cells of the endothelium serve as a physical barrier between the flowing blood and the muscle portion of the artery wall. These cells are tightly interlocked, like tiles on a newly laid countertop. Anything that travels from the blood to the tissues has to pass either through these endothelial cells or through tiny gaps between them.

Just behind the endothelium, inside the artery wall, lies the *media*, a layer of smooth muscle cells that contracts and relaxes on demand. The media squeezes the artery passageway to make it narrower, and relaxes the pressure to let it widen. It does this at the command of the endothelium, which constantly monitors the environment, checking out the blood pressure and other factors. When something isn't quite right, the endothelium sends out certain hormones and mediators to set things straight. For example, if the blood pressure is too high, the endothelium may release nitric oxide (NO for short). The NO tells the media to relax. When the media stops squeezing, the artery gets a little bit wider and the blood pressure falls to a safer level. On the other hand, if the endothelium notices that the blood pressure has dropped too low, it can release various contracting substances that order the media to constrict, thus raising the blood pressure.

In addition to the contraction and dilation of blood vessels, the endothelium helps to control the function of the *platelets*, clotting elements in the blood. It also dictates the thickness and thinness of the blood, how white blood cells stick to the artery walls, the inflammatory process, the growth, thickness, and stiffness of the vascular muscle, and other important factors.

Another important job of the endothelium is to help control *oxidative stress*. Oxidative stress is akin to biochemical thievery. Electrically unbalanced molecules in the body snatch electrons from other substances in order to balance themselves. This may make the thieving molecules "feel better," but the molecules that were "mugged" may not be able to function properly anymore, leading to weakness or destruction of body cells and tissues. The body manufactures *antioxidants* to prevent (or at least control) this kind of damage, and we also absorb various antioxidants from our food. Often, however, the thieving molecules are too much for the body to handle, and we suffer from oxidative stress that can damage the endothelium and encourage hypertension.

In short, the thin layer of cells lining the inside of the arteries acts like a monitoring and correcting station, constantly working to ensure that the blood flows and behaves properly.

> ### BIGGER AND SMALLER PIPES
>
> We've only mentioned arteries and veins, but there are also other kinds of pipes needed to make up the vascular system. There are *arterioles*, which are smaller arteries; *venules*, which are smaller veins; and *capillaries*, the smallest vessels, where the actual exchange of oxygen/nutrients and waste takes place.
>
> Here's how it happens. Freshly oxygenated blood flowing from the heart makes its way through arteries into smaller arterioles, then into the capillaries. The walls of these tiny vessels are composed of only one layer of endothelial cells, making it easy for oxygen and other substances to flow out of the bloodstream and into the cells served by each capillary. Meanwhile, waste products and other substances from the cells cross the endothelium to flow back into the bloodstream. The exchange completed, the oxygen-depleted blood starts its journey back to the heart, flowing from the capillaries into the small venules, then to the larger veins, and finally reaching that all-important muscular pump, the heart.

WHEN THE PIPES ARE PRESSURED

With hypertension, something happens to the endothelium. Just as ocean waves hitting the shore eventually wear away rocks, the constant friction of the blood pushing through the arteries can damage the endothelium. (The endothelium can also be damaged by a variety of other factors, such as high cholesterol, diabetes, aging, or genetic factors that increase the blood pressure.) As the pressure rises within the blood vessels, small cracks or lesions can appear in the endothelium. The body attempts to repair these scratches or cracks by sending in armies of repair and immune system cells, triggering inflammation and trying to set things right. But the repair process is often flawed, and the fixed part of the endothelium often works poorly, a condition called *endothelial dysfunction*.

The damaged area is a prime spot for the formation of *plaque*, a sticky substance made of cholesterol, fat, calcium, and cellular debris. Immune system cells may then burrow through this damaged area into the artery wall, and set up camp there, along with fats and other substances. The upshot of all of this is *atherosclerosis*, a deposition of plaque resulting in constricted, stiffened arteries that can't expand on command to keep blood pressure within normal limits. So damage to the endothelium plays a significant part in bringing on hypertension. In fact, the appearance of endothelial dysfunction often signals the very beginning of vascular disease (e.g., hypertension, atherosclerosis, heart disease, stroke, and other ailments), and can occur *decades* before your blood pressure starts to rise.

ARTERIO VS. ATHERO, EMBOLUS VS. THROMBUS

You may have heard your doctor mention both *arteriosclerosis* and *atherosclerosis*, and wondered if they were the same thing. While their meanings are close, they're not identical. Arteriosclerosis is the thickening, stiffening, and calcification of the artery walls, leading to a decrease in blood supply to an affected tissue. Atherosclerosis is a buildup of plaque in the artery walls, making the walls thick, fibrous, and calcified and reducing the amount of space through which the blood

What Sends Your Blood Pressure Soaring? 21

> can flow. Both are bad news for the arteries and for your blood pressure.
>
> Then there's *thrombus* and *embolus*. A thrombus is a sitting blood clot; it's attached to the interior wall of a blood vessel. An embolus, for our purposes, is a traveling blood clot that eventually gets stuck in a blood vessel.

WHAT IS THE PRESSURE?

Blood pressure (BP) is the amount of force exerted by your blood on the insides of your arteries as the blood is pumped throughout your circulatory system. That pressure is determined by two things:

1. The amount of blood that's pumped from the heart, also known as the *blood volume* or *cardiac output (CO)*. This is the systolic blood pressure, the pressure exerted when your heart contracts. Systolic pressure is expressed as the top part of the fraction (the 120 of 120/80).

2. The resistance offered by the blood vessels as blood is pumped through them, also known as the *systemic vascular resistance (SVR)*. This is the diastolic blood pressure, the pressure exerted when your heart is resting between beats. Diastolic pressure is expressed as the bottom part of the fraction (the 80 of 120/80).

Perhaps the best way to understand blood pressure is to look at the formula we learned in medical school:

$$BP = CO \times SVR$$
(Blood pressure = cardiac output × systemic vascular resistance)

or, to put it in simpler terms:

pressure = force × resistance

In other words, your blood pressure is equal to the *force* of the blood that's being propelled out of your heart multiplied by the *resistance* it encounters from your arteries as the blood is pushed through.

To get a clearer idea of the way blood pressure works, think about a garden hose. If you turn the faucet on just a little, there's not much force available to propel the water, so it trickles out of the hose and falls straight to the ground. But if you turn the faucet up all the way, the water gushes out of the hose and sails through the air for several feet before hitting the ground. That's the force part of the pressure equation.

Now, suppose you turn the faucet on about halfway. There's a good amount of water coming out of the hose, but it only projects about a foot from the mouth of the hose before falling to the ground. If you place your thumb over the end of the hose, however, and then scoot it to the side just slightly so the water is only allowed to come out of a small opening, the water will project halfway across your front lawn. Why? You've provided extra resistance by narrowing the width at the end of the hose, which has increased the pressure. That's the resistance part of the pressure equation.

Within your cardiovascular system, force is a measure of how much blood leaps out of the heart every minute. If you increase the strength or the rate of your heart's pumping action (which happens when you're exercising or you get excited), more blood is pumped and your blood pressure rises.

Inside your body, resistance is an indication of how difficult it is for your blood to travel through your arteries. This is determined by the thickness and stiffness of the muscular layer of the artery and the size of its passageway (the *lumen*). If an artery has thick walls due to plaque buildup or excessive growth of the muscle (*hypertrophy*) or is so stiff that it can't relax properly, it will have a narrow lumen. This makes for less room for the blood to maneuver, increasing resistance and driving up the blood pressure. But an artery with clean, clear walls, or one that can relax and widen on command, will provide plenty of room for the blood to maneuver. Hence, the blood pressure should stay within normal limits.

Another important factor in determining resistance is the thickness (viscosity) of the blood. Thick blood, like sludge, moves more slowly, requiring more force to send it on its way.

CRANKING IT UP

It's a bit of a stretch, but thinking of airplanes and boats can help you understand how force and resistance combine to produce pressure.

An airplane pilot can set the plane to fly at a certain speed (force), say 600 miles per hour. But the sky might be offering resistance in the form of a head wind, which slows the plane down. The pilot may want the plane to zip along at 600 miles per hour, but it's only going 500 miles per hour because of the wind. The airplane's actual speed (pressure) is a combination of force and resistance, or engine speed and head wind.

Similarly, a boat captain can set the craft to sail at a certain engine speed (force), but the craft may have to struggle its way through a current (resistance) flowing the other way.

> The boat's actual speed (pressure) is not the engine speed, but the engine speed minus the speed of the current.

WHAT RAISES THE FORCE?

Your heart will automatically beat harder when you're jogging or you come across a bear in the woods, and that will increase your blood pressure considerably. But this increase *should* happen, so that freshly oxygenated, nutrient-rich blood will be rushed to your tissues, and you'll have the energy to do whatever's necessary. That's not hypertension, even though your blood pressure is high, because once you stop jogging or that bear disappears, your pressure will quickly return to normal. With hypertension, however, your heart is *often or always* working harder than normal and your arteries are *always* narrowed and constricted.

Many factors can send your heart into overdrive:

- *Narrowed arteries*—Your arteries may narrow for several reasons, including plaque buildup, fibrosis, endothelial dysfunction, or in response to messages from your nervous or endocrine systems. When your arteries are narrow, your heart will have to pump harder to push the blood through.
- *Being overweight*—Fat is tissue, just like muscles or organs, and tissue requires a constant blood supply. Some experts estimate that each pound of fat contains about a mile of capillaries, and all those capillaries have to be filled with blood to nourish that fat. That's a lot of extra blood, and a lot of extra pipes to pump the blood through. Just imagine the increased load on your heart if you happen to be carrying forty or fifty extra pounds! Some 60 percent of hypertensive Americans are overweight, which is bad news. The good news is that, in many

cases, just losing ten to twenty pounds can bring blood pressure down to normal levels.

- *Emotional stress*—Anxiety, excitement, fear, anger, and other forms of stress call your body to action through the fight-or-flight mechanism. A burst of adrenaline races to your major organs, increasing your heart rate, blood sugar, blood cholesterol, and blood pressure. This enables you either to fight or to run for your life. Stress not only increases the heart rate, but also the strength of the heart's contractions, both of which magnify the force.
- *Psychological factors*—Aggressive, hard-driving, type A personalities, especially those exhibiting anger, cynicism, and hostility, have increased heart rates and higher cardiac output, resulting in higher blood pressure.
- *Physical stress*—The physical stress experienced during exercise increases cardiac output and drives up blood pressure: That's necessary and temporary. But moderate exercise can actually help *reduce* high blood pressure by making the heart pump more efficiently. It also reduces atherosclerosis, decreases blood fats, and lessens vascular resistance. Yet too much of a good thing *can* be a bad thing. Excessive amounts of activity can increase blood pressure to dangerous levels, especially for those who are usually sedentary or have poorly controlled hypertension. So beware: If you suddenly decide to run a marathon after years of sitting on the couch, your blood pressure might rise to dangerous levels. Other physical stressors, including pain, heat, cold, lack of sleep, and illness, can also push up your blood pressure.
- *Smoking*—You've heard about the dangers of smoking over and over again, but it's particularly bad for your blood pressure. Cigarette smoking revs up your heart rate by increasing tension in the walls of your heart muscle and speeding the

rate of muscular contraction. It also crowds out oxygen with carbon monoxide, meaning there's less oxygen per unit of blood than there should be. This means that you'll need more blood to deliver the same amount of oxygen, which forces your heart to work harder to deliver enough oxygen to the tissues. Smoking increases the risk of atherosclerosis, heart attacks, strokes, and peripheral artery disease (claudication).

- *Hormonal regulators*—Several substances—renin, angiotensin II, endothelin, epinephrine, norepinephrine, cortisol, aldosterone, bradykinin, the prostaglandins, antidiuretic hormone, and many others—play important parts in complex systems that regulate the cardiac output. When these regulators aren't working properly, the blood volume increases, creating more work for the heart.

- *High-sodium diet*—Sodium draws water back into the body from the kidneys, causing fluid retention in sodium-sensitive people. Too much sodium in the diet can also lead to increases in blood pressure in predisposed people via increased blood volume, as well as enlargement of the heart, protein in the urine, kidney disease, and strokes.

- *Pregnancy*—By the latter stages of pregnancy, a woman can have as much as 50 percent more blood flowing through her arteries and veins than she did before she became pregnant. This extra blood volume greatly increases the cardiac output. Normally, the arterioles compensate for this by dilating, so vascular resistance decreases and blood pressure stays within the normal range. But with complications like preeclampsia, toxemia, or eclampsia, there may be moderate to severe increases in blood pressure.

WHAT INCREASES THE RESISTANCE?

Throughout your body, your arteries are constantly in flux, becoming slightly wider or narrower according to what's going on at any given moment. When you're pedaling away furiously on your bicycle, for example, the tiny muscles surrounding the arteries in your legs relax, allowing those arteries to widen and deliver extra blood to your leg muscles. On the other hand, when you plop down on the couch after a big meal, the muscles surrounding the arteries in your legs will actually constrict a bit, while those in your stomach will relax. This makes for less blood delivered to your legs, so the lion's share of blood can be routed toward your digestive system, where it's needed at the moment. The temporary narrowing of certain blood vessels at certain times, therefore, is a healthy and necessary function.

But sometimes blood vessels become permanently narrowed and can't accommodate an increased supply of blood even when it's needed. That's when you get into trouble. Several things can cause this narrowing of the blood vessels (known as *vasoconstriction*), including:

- *Endothelial dysfunction*—When the endothelium is damaged and can't do its job, the blood vessels constrict, become inflamed, and may even leak. Blood vessel walls become thicker, stiffer, and less able to dilate upon command. Clots are more likely to form and there is an increase in oxidative stress.
- *Atherosclerosis*—As you age, your arteries can become narrowed, by the slow buildup of plaque. And they gradually lose their resilience as normal arterial elastic tissue is replaced by fibrous connective tissue (a process called *fibrosis*). As your arteries become narrower and stiffer, they have a harder time dilating.
- *Blood clots*—As the blood flows through plaque-choked

arteries, some of its platelets can get stuck on a protruding piece of plaque, forming a blood clot (*thrombus*). The presence of a clot can severely limit the flow of blood through an artery, or even block it completely. Or the plaque itself can rupture, releasing clotting substances that instantly cause formation of a blood clot. Spontaneous plaque rupture and subsequent clot formation can trigger a heart attack or stroke.

- *Emotional stress*—Stress stimulates the sympathetic nervous system, which in turn constricts your blood vessels, while raising your heart rate and blood pressure. But you don't have to be under severe stress for this to happen. Blood vessel constriction also occurs in response to life's smaller stressors. Accidentally breaking a glass, hearing a loud noise, or just talking to your boss can raise your systolic blood pressure 5 to 10 mm Hg, or more.

- *Psychological factors*—Anger, cynicism, hostility, and other negative emotions promote blood vessel constriction, increasing arterial resistance.

- *Smoking*—Smoking constricts your blood vessels, damages the endothelium, promotes the formation of plaque, and increases the tendency to form blood clots, all of which can drive up blood pressure significantly.

- *Hormonal factors*—Some of the same substances that increase the force of the blood also raise the level of resistance in the arteries, including renin, angiotensin II, endothelin, cortisol, epinephrine, norepinephrine, aldosterone, bradykinin, the prostaglandins, and antidiuretic hormone. When these systems malfunction, the result can be an unnatural constriction of the arteries and an increase in blood pressure.

- *Pregnancy* (with preeclampsia)—Preeclampsia can increase both the force of the blood and the resistance of the blood vessels, sending the blood pressure up to unhealthy levels.

HYPERTENSION IN PREGNANCY

In the average woman, blood pressure actually falls during the first and second trimester, due to the dilation of arterioles and a drop in vascular resistance. But about 10 percent of pregnancies are complicated by hypertension, which can fall into the following categories:

- *Pregnancy-induced hypertension (PIH)*—Also called gestational hypertension, this occurs when the blood pressure rises more than 30/15 mm Hg, or above 140/90 in the last trimester. It usually strikes after the thirty-fifth week of gestation.
- *Chronic hypertension*—Hypertension that existed before twenty weeks gestation.
- *Preeclampsia (also known as toxemia)*—Moderate to severe hypertension that occurs with edema (swelling, usually in the hands and face) and protein in the urine. It occurs after the twentieth week of gestation, more typically after the thirty-sixth week.
- *Eclampsia*—This is preeclampsia plus convulsions and/or coma. It can occur before or during labor, or within forty-eight hours of delivery. Possible effects of untreated preeclampsia or eclampsia are low birth weight, premature delivery, maternal kidney failure, and/or convulsions, and the loss of the baby.

While there is always the potential for danger, with proper medical care, hypertension in pregnancy can be controlled. In most cases, both mother and baby remain healthy.

KINDS OF HYPERTENSION

Most people are surprised to hear that hypertension isn't just a simple case of elevated blood pressure. Yet in over 70 percent of cases, it's an entire metabolic syndrome made up of a complex cluster of abnormalities, including problems with excessive blood clotting, abnormal glucose metabolism, insulin resistance, Type II diabetes, dense LDL ("bad") cholesterol, high triglycerides, and low HDL ("good") cholesterol. The accumulation of belly fat known as apple obesity is also a part of hypertension syndrome. All of these conditions result in damage to the arteries, atherosclerosis, and increased cardiovascular problems. So although the terms "high blood pressure" and "hypertension" are used interchangeably, hypertension is actually a *disease of the blood vessels* involving changes in their structure and function, which is associated with a constellation of other cardiovascular risk factors.

There are two major classifications of hypertension: *essential* (primary or genetic) and *secondary*. Either of these can be mild, moderate, or severe, and may progress to accelerated or malignant hypertension.

- *Essential hypertension* (also known as primary or genetic hypertension) is the most common of the two. In fact, about 90 percent of hypertensives have this form. In essential hypertension, the elevation in blood pressure develops slowly and quietly, but can wield a mighty punch if it remains uncontrolled. No one knows exactly what causes essential hypertension, although the primary reason is genetics. Yet physical, environmental, emotional, and nutritional factors can play important roles in bringing on the disease and making it worse.

- *Secondary hypertension* is a direct result of another disease or condition, including obesity, thyroid or adrenal dysfunction, kidney disease, kidney artery blockages, tumors, and the use of certain medications. This primary disease or condition increases either the resistance of the blood vessels or the amount of blood being pushed through the system, resulting in high blood pressure. Luckily, once the primary problem is corrected, the hypertension usually vanishes. Causes of secondary hypertension include:

- Acromegaly (gigantism)
- Coarctation of the aorta (narrowing of the aorta)
- Cushing's syndrome (a metabolic disorder resulting in excessive production of the steroid hormone cortisol)
- Decongestants
- Hyperparathyroidism (too much parathyroid hormone)
- Kidney disease
- Licorice intoxication (from eating too much licorice)
- Oral contraceptives (which push the blood pressure up an average of 5 percent after seven years of use)
- Pheochromocytoma (vascular tumor)
- Primary aldosteronism (too much aldosterone, the hormone that regulates sodium and potassium balance in the blood)
- Renovascular hypertension (high blood pressure resulting from disease of the arteries to the kidneys)
- Sleep apnea (temporary stoppage of breathing during sleep)
- Thyroid disease (hyperthyroidism, hypothyroidism)
- Various pain relievers, including the nonsteroidal medications (such as aspirin, ibuprofen, and COX-2 inhibitors)
- Certain toxins, including alcohol and cocaine
- Diet pills (such as ephedra)

- *Accelerated and malignant hypertension* are medical emergencies that can develop from either essential or secondary hypertension, particularly if they're untreated. Accelerated hypertension is a sudden rise in blood pressure in a patient who has essential hypertension. Malignant hypertension is an extremely dangerous form of the disease characterized by a very high diastolic pressure (over 120 mm Hg), blurred vision, severe headaches, visual disturbances, and seizures. It can result in congestive heart failure, heart attack, stroke, and/or acute renal failure (inability of the kidneys to function properly), and in some cases, it can be fatal. Emergency lifesaving treatment to reduce blood pressure and attack the underlying cause of this disease is crucial.

WHITE COAT HYPERTENSION

There's another fairly common kind of hypertension called *white coat hypertension.* This is blood pressure that rises to unhealthy levels when you're in your doctor's office, at the hospital, or when you're stressed or anxious, but is normal at other times.

No, it doesn't happen because you're allergic to your doctor, or because of that funny smell so many hospitals have. It's due to tension. You know that your blood pressure is being checked, and you know that a bad reading could mean you're seriously ill, so you get scared and your pressure rises. But after you've been sitting quietly for a while and you've been reassured by your doctor that there's nothing to worry about, a repeat reading may show that your pressure is fine. Or maybe your pressure will remain elevated while you're in the

> office or at the hospital, but will stay within normal limits during a twenty-four-hour ambulatory blood pressure monitoring (which measures your pressure off and on while you're going through a typical day).
>
> You might think that white coat hypertension isn't a serious problem—just a case of the jitters that temporarily skews body chemistry. But some studies suggest it's a problem worthy of concern because it's linked to changes in vascular resistance, elevated blood fats, increased LDL (bad) cholesterol, insulin resistance, and other problems, any of which can increase cardiovascular risk.

SO WHAT'S SO TERRIBLE ABOUT HIGH BLOOD PRESSURE?

Aside from the malignant form, why are we so afraid of elevated blood pressure? So what if things are running in overdrive inside your pipes? In fact, if you hadn't always heard that high blood pressure was bad for your health, you might think it was a sign of a strong, healthy heart. After all, with hypertension your heart is beating hard and getting a workout, even when you're just sitting around doing nothing. Isn't all that exercise bound to make it even stronger?

Unfortunately, the reverse is true. Hypertension pounds away at some of your most vital organs, including your arteries, heart, brain, kidneys, and eyes, and if left untreated it can kill you. Let's take a look at how untreated hypertension wreaks havoc on some of your vital organs.

Hypertension Damages the Vascular System

Hypertension attacks and damages the blood vessels by eroding their lining, making them less resilient, and depositing a sticky plaque that narrows their passageways or chokes them off completely. The major ways in which hypertension attacks the vascular system include:

- *Endothelial dysfunction*—The sheer stress of the blood pounding away at the endothelium scrambles the single layer of cells lining the inner artery walls, leaving them disorganized and unable to perform their biochemical chores. As a result, blood vessels no longer dilate and constrict properly, platelets begin to clump, blood clots form, inflammation reigns, and both blood vessel leakage and oxidative stress increase.
- *Atherosclerosis*—As you grow older and as the endothelium suffers more and more damage, the arterial walls accumulate a layer of plaque. In addition, they become thick, fiber-fouled (fibrotic), and calcified, which narrows their passageways and makes them less resilient. Although this process happens to a certain extent in everyone as they age, it is accelerated by hypertension.
- *Aortic aneurysm*—The constant, excessive pounding of blood through the body's largest artery can eventually cause its inner lining to tear, and its outer and middle layers to separate. In other words, the aorta can begin to split lengthwise from the inside. If it should continue to split through all three layers and rupture, death could occur in less than an hour due to massive internal blood loss and shock.

Hypertension Damages the Heart

Left untreated, hypertension greatly increases your chances of developing heart disease, suffering a cardiac complication, or dying at an early age. In fact, for every 10 mm Hg rise in mean arterial pressure, there is a 40 percent rise in cardiovascular risk. Hypertension damages the heart in two major ways, by overworking it (leading to heart failure) and by clogging up its own arteries (leading to a heart attack).

- *Heart failure*—As the arteries throughout the body become constricted and/or plaque-filled, the heart must work harder to push the blood through the circulatory system. Under pressure from this increased workload, it gradually enlarges and becomes stiffer, a condition known as *cardiomegaly*. This makes the heart less efficient; soon it becomes weak, flabby, and unable to meet the body's demands.

When the heart becomes so overworked that it can't do its job properly, it begins to fail. Typically, the left side of the heart is in trouble in hypertensives, causing a condition known as *left-ventricular hypertrophy*. Shortness of breath, prolonged circulation time, water retention, and fatigue are common symptoms. Right-sided heart failure can trigger swelling of the legs and ankles, enlargement of the liver, and distention of the jugular vein.

- *Coronary artery disease*—Approximately 80 percent of hypertensive patients also have low levels of HDL ("good") cholesterol and high levels of total cholesterol, triglycerides, LDL ("bad") cholesterol, and VLDL (very low density lipoprotein, another "bad" kind of cholesterol). Over time, this increase in blood fats and decrease in HDL can promote plaque formation inside the heart's own arteries, a condition known as *coronary heart disease*. Combine that with endothelial dysfunction, abnormal constriction of the blood vessels, and the supercharged force of the blood pounding away at the artery walls and you've got a recipe for *angina* (suffocating pain in the chest, shoulder, or arm indicating a lack of oxygen to the heart) or *myocardial infarction* (a heart attack).

LIFE EXPECTANCY AND BLOOD PRESSURE

The higher your blood pressure, the shorter your life expectancy. Here's the life expectancy of a thirty-five-year-old man according to his blood pressure reading:

Blood Pressure (mm Hg)	Life Expectancy (years)
120/80	76
130/90	67½
140/95	62½
150/100	55

Hypertension Damages the Brain

Hypertension is a major cause of disability and the number one cause of stroke. It causes strokes by weakening and wearing away at the lining of the brain arteries, and choking those arteries with plaque. The damaged linings provide a perfect site for plaque deposition and the formation of blood clots. A stroke can happen in one of three ways: A brain artery can become completely choked off, a free-floating clot can block it, or it may simply rupture. The result of all three is the same: a lack of oxygen to the area of the brain served by the artery, and the death of brain tissue in that area. One out of three strokes is fatal, and hypertension is the third leading cause of death in this country.

> ### IT'S NOT JUST ALZHEIMER'S
>
> Seniors, and even Baby Boomers, are terrified of Alzheimer's disease, that "brain eraser" that robs so many Americans of their minds. But the number one cause of dementia in the United States may actually be hypertension, which causes a condition called *vascular dementia*. This disease of the small arteries in the brain leads to memory loss, as well as cognitive, behavioral, and emotional abnormalities similar to those seen in Alzheimer's disease.
>
> Vascular dementia is primarily caused by hypertension, although elevated cholesterol, diabetes mellitus (Type I or Type II), and high levels of homocysteine in the blood can also be to blame.
>
> The diagnosis of vascular dementia is made on the basis of the patient's symptoms plus an abnormal CT (CAT scan) or MRI (magnetic resonance imaging) of the brain showing "white matter disease" (the death of brain tissue due to atherosclerosis, thrombosis, vasoconstriction, or other problems with the brain's small arteries).

Hypertension Damages the Kidneys

There's a kind of reciprocal relationship between hypertension and the kidneys. Hypertension can cause kidney disease, and kidney disease can cause hypertension.

The kidneys are key to health; they perform the extremely important function of filtering wastes from the blood, then channeling it into the urine for excretion. But uncontrolled high blood pressure brings on premature atherosclerosis to the blood vessels in the kidneys, decreasing their supply of oxygen and nutrients. As a result, they become less efficient. Toxins build up in the blood, leading to a condition called *uremia*, which can progress to kidney failure. Unable to cleanse itself, the body essentially begins to drown in its own waste.

That's how hypertension triggers kidney disease. But it also works the other way. The kidneys play an important role in controlling blood pressure through the complex renin-angiotensin-aldosterone system. In a nutshell, the kidneys release the enzyme renin, which causes a chain reaction resulting in an increase in blood volume, coupled with the constriction of blood vessels: the perfect conditions for elevated blood pressure. It works like this:

• The kidneys produce *renin*, which flows through the bloodstream.

• Renin acts on a polypeptide called *angiotensinogen*, which is converted to a substance called *angiotensin I*.

• Angiotensin I is then converted to *angiotensin II*, a powerful blood vessel constrictor. The conversion is accomplished via angiotensin-converting enzyme (ACE), which is found in all arteries, as well as in the lungs.

• Angiotensin II narrows the blood vessels and causes local damage to the arteries, triggering endothelial dysfunction, vascular growth, clots, oxidative stress, among other disorders. It also stimulates the secretion of a substance called *aldosterone*.

• Aldosterone holds on to sodium and water in the kidneys that normally would be excreted. It also damages the arteries in ways similar to angiotensin II.

- Sodium and water are returned to the bloodstream, increasing blood volume.
- The upshot is this: An increase in blood volume plus an increase in blood vessel constriction equals an increase in blood pressure.

In a normal body, this chain reaction is only kicked into gear when blood volume or sodium is low or when the body is dehydrated. But if it goes into action when the blood pressure is normal or, even worse, when it's already high, you've got problems. In other words, if your kidneys malfunction and send out the wrong enzyme at the wrong time, your blood pressure is heading upward.

Hypertension Damages the Eyes

Using an ophthalmoscope, a doctor can often see evidence of hypertension in the retina, the delicate membrane inside the eye that receives the image formed by the lens, then sends it to the brain via the optic nerve. Narrowing of the arterioles, a stiffened artery compressing a vein (*AV nicking*), protein from damaged arteries leaking into the retina (*exudates*), hemorrhages, and edema, among other things, can indicate the presence and the severity of hypertension.

Hypertension takes its toll on the eyes in the same way it does elsewhere. The excess force caused by the pounding of the blood upsets the endothelium of the small arteries that supply the retina with blood. This causes a narrowing and thickening of the arteries, a decrease in the blood supply to the retina, and atherosclerosis. Eventually, tiny ruptures can occur in capillaries that serve the retina, fat deposits can accumulate, and the optic nerve can swell. Left untreated, severe cases of high blood pressure can result in blindness.

WHAT WILL MAKE YOU MORE LIKELY TO DEVELOP HYPERTENSION?

Hypertension is *not* an equal opportunity disease; it definitely has its preferred targets. Some risk factors for hypertension may simply be part of your makeup and can't be altered. But many of them can be changed, and doing so can make a big difference to your health.

Risk Factors You Can't Change

- *Age*—Your risk of developing high blood pressure rises as you age. In fact, 50 percent of adults over the age of sixty, and 80 percent of those over the age of seventy, have hypertension (especially systolic hypertension). This is most likely due to the age-related progression of atherosclerosis, but may also be due to being overweight, lack of exercise, poor nutrition and diet, and/or a general decrease in kidney function.
- *Genetics*—If one of your parents had high blood pressure, you have a 25 percent chance of developing the disease yourself. If both your parents had high blood pressure, your odds rise to 50 percent. The risk increases if both parents, or a parent and a sibling, have hypertension. The genetic link is particularly noticeable in those who develop hypertension before the age of fifty, who are 3.8 times more likely to have a family history of the disease.
- *Race*—African-Americans are a favorite target of hypertension: The disease strikes one out of three African-Americans, as opposed to one out of four Caucasians. It also tends to occur at a younger age in African-Americans, and generally produces more serious results at every blood pressure level, with a higher illness and death rate than you'll find in any other race. In

1999, the hypertension death rate per 100,000 people was 46.8 for African-American males and 40.3 for African-American females, as opposed to 12.8 for white males and 12.8 for white females.

- *Sex*—Up until the age of sixty, women are less likely than men to develop high blood pressure, but after age sixty, women take the lead, especially in systolic hypertension. However, female hypertensives seem to fare better than their male counterparts, suffering from fewer cardiovascular problems in the long run.

Risk Factors You Can Change

- *Alcohol abuse*—Excessive alcohol consumption can progressively increase both systolic and diastolic blood pressure, and in some people may actually be the cause of hypertension. It's best to eliminate alcohol completely if you have hypertension, but some people can tolerate small amounts of alcohol with no adverse effects. If you drink, your daily limit should be less than 24 ounces of beer *or* 10 ounces of wine *or* 2 ounces of hard liquor. (Notice I say "or," not "and.")
- *Drug use*—Certain kinds of prescription, over-the-counter, and recreational drugs can increase blood pressure. Ask your doctor if any of the prescription or nonprescription drugs you are taking may be pushing up your blood pressure. As for recreational drugs, avoid them entirely!

Be especially wary of:
- Appetite suppressants and amphetamine-like drugs
- Cocaine
- Corticosteroids such as cortisone and steroids
- Cyclosporine, which suppresses the immune system

- Decongestants such as pseudoephedrine
- Ephedra (a herb, also known as Ma huang)
- Erythropoietin, a medicine for anemia
- MAO inhibitors and phenothiazines such as antidepressants and antipsychotics
- Nonsteroidal anti-inflammatories (NSAIDs), such as aspirin and ibuprofen, which increase sodium and water retention and induce vasoconstriction
- COX-2 inhibitors, the new medicines for osteoarthritis, which can increase the blood pressure just as the NSAIDs do, although perhaps not as much
- Oral contraceptives, which activate the renin-angiotensin-aldosterone system

• *Poor diet*—High intakes of sodium, saturated fat, trans fatty acids, refined carbohydrates, sugar, and possibly caffeine can all contribute to hypertension. (We'll talk about changing your diet to reduce your blood pressure in Chapters 5 and 6.)

• *Lack of exercise*—Regular exercise lowers blood pressure, blood fats, blood glucose, vascular resistance, and risk of cardiovascular disease. It also improves endothelial function and coronary artery blood flow, increases lean muscle mass, and decreases weight and total body fat.

• *Obesity*—Obesity in early adulthood, between the ages of twenty and thirty, significantly increases the risk of developing hypertension later on. Luckily, just losing some of those extra pounds is one of the most effective ways to reduce elevated blood pressure, lessen the heart's workload, and increase overall cardiac efficiency.

• *Smoking*—Simply tossing away the cigarettes, cigars, pipes, snuff, and chewing tobacco will lead to improvements in your cardiovascular system within one year, no matter what your age.

Risk Factors You May (or May Not) Be Able to Change

- *Education and income*—For reasons we do not entirely understand, people with more education and higher incomes tend to have less hypertension than their counterparts with fewer years of schooling and lower incomes.
- *Emotional stress*—Physical exercise, relaxation, meditation, and other physical and mental methods of stress release are vitally important for lowering blood pressure and maintaining physical and mental health. (We'll talk more about this in Chapters 7 and 8.)
- *Various diseases or conditions that bring on secondary hypertension*—Secondary hypertension is the result of another condition or disease and is found most often in children. Hypertension stemming from another source can't be treated successfully until the primary disease or condition is addressed.

ARE THERE ANY OBVIOUS SIGNS OF HYPERTENSION?

The best way to determine whether you've got hypertension is to get regular, accurate, and repeated blood pressure readings at your doctor's office. While there are usually no symptoms in the early stages of hypertension, as it becomes more severe you may experience one or more of the following:

- Hypertension headache (usually occurs at the back of the head just above the neck, and feels worse when you first awaken in the morning)
- Dizziness
- Blackouts
- Blurred vision

- Chest pain
- Heart palpitations
- Ringing in the ears
- Numbness or weakness on one side
- Water retention in the extremities
- Shortness of breath
- Fatigue
- Nosebleed
- Overall weakness
- Excessive urination at night

Naturally, should you experience any of these symptoms, you'll need to see your physician immediately for a thorough evaluation. They are indications of serious trouble that warrant prompt medical attention, whether or not they are related to hypertension.

Chapter 3

The Multifaceted Solution

Several years ago I decided to delve into the alternative scientific literature, hoping to find a few vitamins or minerals that might improve my own heart health and slow the effects of Father Time. Although I expected to find some information on these topics, I was amazed to find over 1,000 studies describing the ways in which vitamins, minerals, herbs, antioxidants, and other nutraceuticals could reduce elevated blood pressure—sometimes as well as standard medicines.

Excited by the possibility of new treatments for my patients, I expanded my search, casting my net wider in an attempt to learn all I could about the effects of food, nutraceuticals, and supplements on hypertension. Here, in short, is what I found:

1. Consuming excessive amounts of certain nutrients, like sodium, saturated fats, and trans fatty acids, can contribute to the development and worsening of hypertension.

2. Other nutrients can prevent, control, and treat hypertension, such as vitamin C, potassium, magnesium, and coenzyme Q_{10}. They do so in various ways, mainly by relaxing the

arteries, protecting the lining of the blood vessels, and disarming dangerous oxidants.

3. In general, whole foods and whole food concentrates (concentrated food products made from the entire vegetable or fruit) are superior to individual components (such as magnesium supplements). In other words, it's usually better to get your vitamin C from oranges, lemons, grapefruit, papaya, guava, red peppers, cantaloupe, or black currants, rather than from pills.

4. However, the selective use of individual vitamins, antioxidants, or other nutraceuticals in supplement form can be very helpful. These individual components should be used to *complement* rather than replace good nutrition.

That's the basic idea. This chapter is a slimmed-down, reader-friendly version of my findings, briefly explaining how several nutraceuticals combat hypertension, listing some foods that contain them, and giving recommended amounts. For a more detailed discussion of this topic, see the Appendix.

By the way, this chapter only looks at the *helpful* substances in food. For a discussion of the *harmful* substances in food, foods as a whole, and effective diets for lowering blood pressure, see Chapters 5 and 6.

DOCTOR DRUG TALK

In this chapter we're going to be comparing the health-enhancing effects of some foodstuffs and supplements to those of hypertension medicines. In order to understand these comparisons, you need to know a little bit of doctor jargon.

This is not a complete listing or discussion of the various

antihypertensive drugs, just a brief rundown of the ones mentioned in this chapter. The complete discussion of medicines for hypertension is found in Chapter 9.

- *Angiotensin-converting enzyme inhibitors,* known as ACE inhibitors or ACEIs, help reduce blood pressure by interfering with the angiotensin-converting enzyme (ACE). This enzyme is part of the renin-angiotensin-aldosterone system, which causes the constriction of muscles surrounding the arteries, raising the blood pressure.
- *Angiotensin II receptor blockers,* known as ARBs, also interfere with the renin-angiotensin-aldosterone system.
- *Beta blockers* reduce blood pressure by slowing the heart rate, reducing cardiac output, and inhibiting the body's ability to raise blood pressure through the renin-angiotensin-aldosterone system.
- *Calcium channel blockers,* known as CCBs, inhibit the movement of calcium into the smooth muscle wrapped around the arteries, allowing the muscles to relax and the arteries to dilate.
- *Central alpha antagonists* work to dampen certain effects of the sympathetic nervous system, thus reducing vascular resistance and lowering blood pressure.
- *Diuretics* flush excess fluid out of the body, or relax artery muscle.
- *Vasodilators* encourage the arteries to relax and open wider.

NUTRACEUTICALS AGAINST HYPERTENSION

We'll begin with a look at potassium, calcium, and magnesium, minerals that have long been recommended by the medical establishment to help control hypertension. Then we'll move on to examine some of the more newly recognized substances such as omega-3 and omega-6 fatty acids, olive oil, vitamin C, coenzyme Q_{10}, celery, garlic and its active ingredient allicin, seaweed, vitamin E, vitamin D, vitamin B_6, zinc, taurine, lycopene, L-carnitine, alpha lipoic acids, flavonoids, N-acetyl cysteine, L-arginine, hawthorn berry, fiber, and guava fruit. Finally, I'll briefly mention some herbs that *may* be helpful.

Note: Just as you should consult with your physician before changing your medication regimen, you should also check with him or her before you begin or stop taking any supplements, or change the doses.

A FEW ABBREVIATIONS

In this chapter you'll see a few abbreviations we use to describe quantities of vitamins, minerals, and nutraceuticals. They are:

mg = milligrams
mcg = micrograms
MEq = milliequivalents
IU = International Units

POTASSIUM

Way back in 1928, a report was published suggesting that a high potassium intake could reduce elevated blood pressure.[1]

This early observation was confirmed by population studies showing that there was less hypertension in large groups of people who had high intakes of potassium, compared to large groups who consumed less potassium.[2] There are also large-scale surveys showing that this holds true for individuals, not just large groups.[3]

Interestingly, the potassium-hypertension link appears to be strongest among people who are also eating a high-sodium diet. What's the link between potassium and sodium? The two work in opposition within the body to perform many functions, including regulation of the blood pressure. This means that these two minerals must be balanced: Too much sodium compared to potassium can tip the scales in favor of hypertension, while too little sodium compared to potassium can leave you with low blood pressure.

The average American has a potassium-to-sodium ratio of 1:2, or less.[4] That is, for each unit of potassium they consume, they take in two units of sodium. We're taking in much less potassium (compared to sodium) than did the cave people who lived back during the Paleolithic era: Our hearty ancestors consumed a potassium-to-sodium ratio of 5:1.

Numerous population, observational, and clinical studies have demonstrated that blood pressure falls when dietary potassium is increased.[5] And it doesn't take much to accomplish a lot. In hypertensives, supplementing with 60 to 120 mEq (or 2,400 to 4,800 mg) of potassium per day leads to an average drop of 4.4 mm Hg in the systolic pressure, and 2.5 mm Hg in the diastolic pressure. A high potassium intake reduces the blood pressure most effectively in people who are taking in large amounts of sodium, have salt-sensitive hypertension, severe hypertension, and/or are of African-American or Chinese descent.[6]

> ## Potassium Facts
>
> Potassium is the third most abundant element in the body, with most of it residing inside the body cells. Independent of its effects on hypertension, the mineral can also reduce the incidence of heart attacks and stroke.
>
> *Duties:* Potassium has several duties in the body, including helping the muscles and nervous system work properly. It also works with sodium and chloride to distribute fluids properly throughout the body.
>
> *Deficiency:* Although we rarely see serious deficiencies of potassium, you may find yourself suffering from a lesser deficiency if, for example, you have recently suffered from prolonged bouts of diarrhea or vomiting, you've severely restricted your calorie intake, or you use diuretics.
>
> *Excess:* If you're getting all your potassium from foods, you don't have to worry about developing potassium toxicity (overdose), unless you have kidney disease. However, it is possible to take in too much of the mineral via supplements, so be careful not to exceed 100 mEq (4,000 mg) via supplements per day.

I recommended a potassium intake of 100 mEq (4,000 mg) or more per day, with the bulk of it in food form. You can find potassium in a number of foods, including green leafy vegetables, nuts, papayas, dates, bananas, cantaloupes, guavas, and oranges, or in pure potassium chloride salt substitutes.

CALCIUM

The calcium-hypertension link begins with water—specifically, hard water containing calcium and other minerals. Researchers noted that populations drinking hard water had less cardiovascular disease than those sipping soft water, which contains less calcium and more sodium. They also noted that among large groups of people, more calcium in the diet was linked to lower blood pressure, as well as a reduced risk of developing hypertension. Indeed, people consuming greater than 800 mg of calcium per day have a 23 percent lower risk of developing hypertension, compared to those consuming less than 400 mg per day.

Recently, the calcium-hypertension question was examined in a meta-analysis,[7] a study that pooled the results of several other studies. The authors found that giving calcium supplements to hypertensive patients lowered their systolic blood pressure an average of 4.3 mm Hg, and their diastolic by 1.5 mm Hg.

Yet the results on supplemental calcium are mixed. Some studies show it effectively reduces blood pressure, while others do not. Why the discrepancy? It depends on who's participating in the study. It may also depend on the type and amount of calcium consumed and its relationship to other minerals, such as sodium, potassium, and magnesium. Certain hypertensives respond well to supplemental calcium, including African-Americans, the elderly, pregnant women, menopausal women, people with salt-sensitive hypertension or low-renin hypertension, those who consume a lot of sodium, and those with Type II diabetes. Folks who don't fall into any of these categories may not respond well. If you look only at studies involving the good responders listed above, supplemental calcium appears to be a winner. For even greater reliability, though, try increasing your intake of calcium-containing foods rather than simply taking a calcium supplement.

CALCIUM FACTS

Calcium is the most abundant element in the body. Most of that calcium can be found in your bones and teeth, with just small amounts in your blood, muscles, nerves, and elsewhere.

Duties: Calcium is vital for the growth and maintenance of strong bones and teeth. It also helps with blood clotting, muscle contraction, and the function of certain enzyme systems. In addition, calcium helps keep the heart beating regularly.

Deficiency: In children, a diet severely lacking in calcium leads to rickets, with its characteristic soft bones and poor growth. Adults lacking calcium can develop a similar disease called osteomalacia. Osteoporosis, in which the bones become thinner, more porous, and subject to fracture, can also result from a long-term lack of calcium. Muscle cramps can be an early sign of calcium deficiency.

Excess: Most people can consume a large amount of calcium—over 2,000 mg per day from foods and supplements—without suffering ill effects. It is possible, however, to take in too much. Signs of excess include fatigue, muscle weakness, kidney stones, and other problems.

I recommended an intake of calcium of between 1,000 and 1,500 mg per day. You can find calcium in a number of foods, including milk, yogurt, cheese, canned salmon or sardines (with the bones), almonds, cantaloupes, and broccoli.

VITAMIN D

Many population and experimental studies have linked the active form of vitamin D (vitamin D_3) to blood pressure. These studies have shown that when the amount of vitamin D drops too far, the blood pressure rises—and so does the VLDL ("bad") cholesterol. The body's ability to clear fat from the blood following a fatty meal slows as well.

We haven't yet mapped out all the ways in which the vitamin lowers pressure, but we do know that D affects the cell membranes (walls), and aids in the absorption, use, and excretion of calcium. But because vitamin D appears to reduce elevated blood pressure through its relationship to calcium, it's been difficult to tell how much of the reduction is due directly to vitamin D, and how much is due to calcium. Still, it's clear that vitamin D has positive effects on blood pressure. It may even make calcium more potent, as suggested by a study of 148 elderly, hypertensive women with low levels of vitamin D. Giving them 1,200 mg of calcium reduced their blood pressure. But giving them 1,200 mg of calcium *plus* 800 IU of vitamin D_3 reduced their systolic blood pressure an additional *9.3 percent*.[8]

D Facts

Vitamin D is sometimes called the "sunshine vitamin" because it can be manufactured in the skin when the body is exposed to sunlight.

> *Duties:* Vitamin D is necessary for healthy bones, muscles, and cells. It also helps the body absorb and use phosphorus and calcium.
>
> *Deficiency:* A deficiency of vitamin D can lead to rickets in children, causing bowed legs, a bent spine, and weak muscles. The adult form of this disease is called osteomalacia. A deficiency in vitamin D can also lead to osteoporosis, tooth decay, and nervous system disorders.
>
> *Excess:* The body tends to hang on to vitamin D since it's stored in fat tissue, so don't take more than the recommended amount without consulting your physician. Signs of excess include headaches, nausea, digestive problems, weakness, and irreversible kidney damage. Excessive amounts of vitamin D can also interfere with the body's ability to regulate levels of calcium in the bones and soft tissues.

I recommend a vitamin D intake of 200 to 400 IU per day, depending on age, gender, kidney function, and other factors. You can find vitamin D in fortified milk, cod liver oil, and other fish oils. Cheese and other dairy products are not necessarily good sources of vitamin D since they're not always made from fortified milk.

MAGNESIUM

The mineral magnesium plays a key role in maintaining normal blood pressure levels. It does so by helping to regulate the systolic and diastolic pressure, as well as the ability of the arteries to relax and squeeze upon demand. Magnesium is an essential co-factor in the series of biochemical steps leading to the creation of prostaglandin E_1, a powerful vasodilator. Furthermore, it regulates the amount of sodium, calcium, and potassium found within the cells—three minerals that play key roles in maintaining healthy blood pressure levels. Magnesium also serves as a co-factor in the production of ATP (adenosine triphosphate), the basic energy source for all body cells.

Many population studies have shown that there is an inverse relationship between the amount of magnesium consumed in the diet and blood pressure. That is, the more magnesium consumed in the form of food, the lower the blood pressure. Between 500 and 1,000 mg of dietary magnesium per day seems to be the optimal amount for lowering elevated pressure.

Magnesium supplements can also be beneficial. In a recent study,[9] sixty people suffering from essential hypertension saw their blood pressure levels fall significantly when they were given 500 mg of supplemental magnesium per day. And in a 1994 study,[10] ninety-one middle-aged and elderly women with mild to moderate hypertension were given either a magnesium preparation containing 485 mg of magnesium, or a placebo, for six months. In those taking the magnesium, systolic pressure fell by 2.7 mm Hg, and diastolic by 3.4 mm Hg.

While not all the magnesium–blood pressure studies have yielded such positive results, we can safely conclude that for many people magnesium helps lower blood pressure and is likely to be more valuable when consumed with calcium and potassium rather than as a stand-alone supplement.

MAGNESIUM FACTS

More than half of the magnesium in your body is found in your bones and teeth; slightly more than 25 percent is in your

> liver, muscles, and other soft tissues; a small amount is in your blood and other body fluids.
>
> *Duties:* The body uses magnesium to manufacture protein, as well as to convert protein, fat, and carbohydrates into energy. This mineral also helps detoxify the body and keep the blood from clotting unnecessarily. Magnesium may play a role in regulating glucose tolerance, thereby warding off diabetes.
>
> *Deficiency:* A severe magnesium deficiency can trigger fatigue, confusion, the jitters, muscle spasms, and irregular heartbeat.
>
> *Excess:* Signs of magnesium excess include mental confusion, muscle weakness, and difficulty breathing.

I recommend a magnesium intake of 500 to 1,000 mg per day, primarily from foods. You can find magnesium in a number of foods, including peas, beans, whole grain breads, avocados, dry-roasted almonds, lima beans, dark green vegetables, nuts, and seafood.

A SPECIAL NOTE ON CALCIUM, POTASSIUM, MAGNESIUM, AND SODIUM

Calcium, magnesium, potassium, and a reduced amount of sodium work in concert to optimize blood pressure. And each influences the actions of the others. For example, low magnesium will cause low potassium, so until the missing magnesium is replaced, taking potassium alone will not increase blood potassium levels. And if you want to reduce blood pressure, taking more calcium, potassium, and magnesium together, coupled with a low sodium intake, will be more effective than doing any of these things by itself. When you think of any of these minerals, think of all four.

PROTEIN

Several observational and population studies looking at Japanese, American, and British groups have linked a high protein intake to a reduction in blood pressure.[11] But the type of protein is very important, for animal protein is less effective than nonanimal protein.[12] Vegetable protein, soy and beans, and whey are best, but protein in the form of meat from lean or wild animals, such as range-fed cattle, is a good alternative. It typically contains less saturated fat and more omega-3 and omega-6 fatty acids than other kinds of animal protein.

The Intersalt Study, a large-scale international observational program involving 10,020 men and women in thirty-two countries, supported the idea that higher dietary protein intake has positive effects on blood pressure. The study found that those consuming 30 percent above the average protein intake had lower blood pressures than in those eating 30 percent less than the average protein intake. The average systolic BP was 3.0 mm Hg lower, and the average diastolic BP was 2.5 mm Hg lower.

Studies have looked at protein from a number of sources, including meat, soy, fermented milk supplemented with whey protein concentrate, and sardine muscle. Their positive effects on blood pressure are due, in part, to the protein itself, which may behave like an ACE inhibitor drug, and may induce the body to excrete sodium via the urine (*natriuresis*). Other substances found in conjunction with the protein source probably also play a role. For example, milk contains good amounts of whey protein, as well as such antihypertensive ingredients as vitamin D, calcium, and potassium.

I recommend a protein intake of 1.0 to 1.2 grams per kilogram of body weight (varies with exercise). If you weigh 150 pounds, that works out to 68 to 82 grams of protein per day, approximately the amount found in 6 ounces of meat plus 3 glasses of skim milk plus 2 slices of whole wheat or whole grain bread. Another way to look at it is this: Protein should account for 30 percent of the calories you consume every day. But remember, nonanimal sources of protein, such as soy and beans, are best. Meat from lean or wild animals, such as range-fed cattle, is an acceptable second choice.

Other particularly helpful forms of protein include:

- Hydrolyzed whey protein—30 grams per day
- Soy protein (preferably fermented)—30 grams per day
- Hydrolyzed wheat germ isolate—2 to 4 grams per day
- Sardine muscle concentrate extract—3 mg per day

OMEGA-3 POLYUNSATURATED FATTY ACIDS

You've probably heard the term "omega-3 fatty acids" bandied about, and quite likely noticed that it seemed to be used interchangeably with "fish oil." They're really not one in the same, although they're close. And studies have shown that both can help reduce blood pressure in people with mild hypertension.

But before I jump into a discussion of the effects of omega-3 polyunsaturated fatty acids (PUFAs, for short) on hypertension, let me define a few terms: *Fatty acids* are the major components of the fat molecule, just as amino acids are the building blocks of protein. If you look at a diagram of a fatty

The Multifaceted Solution

acid in a textbook, you'll see that it's built around a line of carbon atoms. The carbons are lined up like boxcars in a train, and each has four arms: one to the front, one to the rear, one to the right and one to the left. With its rear arm, it holds on to the carbon behind, with its front arm it grasps the carbon ahead. With its left and right arms it holds on to two hydrogen atoms, one out to either side. If every side arm of every carbon in the line is holding on to a hydrogen atom, we call the fatty acid *saturated*. It's all filled up and can't possibly hold any more hydrogens.

But sometimes, two adjacent carbon atoms in the line each let go of a hydrogen atom. Then, with their free arms, they grab hold of each other, forming what we call a double bond. We call this kind of fatty acid *unsaturated*, because it's not holding on to as many hydrogens as it might. If just a single pair of carbons forms a double bond, it's called a *monounsaturated fatty acid (MUFA)*. If more than one pair form a double bond, it's called a *polyunsaturated fatty acid (PUFA)*.

The location of the double bond makes a difference in the characteristics of the fat, so we note that in the name of that fat. If the double bond occurs after the third carbon from the omega end, the fatty acid is called an *omega-3 fatty acid*. If it occurs after the sixth carbon from the omega end, it's called an *omega-6 fatty acid*.

The kind of fats that can help lower blood pressure the most and improve overall heart health are the omega-3 fatty acids. Since some of the best sources of omega 3s are fish, some people use the term "omega-3 fatty acids" interchangeably with "fish" or "fish oil." This is incorrect, however, since there are also nonfish sources of omega 3s, such as green soybeans, butternuts, green leafy vegetables, flaxseed oil, canola oil, walnuts, and Brazil nuts.

Here are two simplified drawings of fatty acids. C is a carbon atom, H is a hydrogen atom, O is an oxygen atom, a vertical or horizontal dash indicates a bond, and a double vertical or horizontal dash indicates a double bond.

This is a saturated fatty acid, for all of the carbon atoms in the main body of the fatty acid are attached to two hydrogen atoms, one above and one below.

```
    H   H   H   H   H   H   H   H   H   O
    |   |   |   |   |   |   |   |   |   ||
H - C - C - C - C - C - C - C - C - C - C - O - H
    |   |   |   |   |   |   |   |   |
    H   H   H   H   H   H   H   H   H
```

Here's an unsaturated fatty acid: At least two of the carbon atoms have each let go of a hydrogen atom. Since the first carbon atom to have let go is in the third position, this is an omega-3 fatty acid.

```
    H   H   H   H   H   H   H   H   H   O
    |   |   |   |   |   |   |   |   |   ||
H - C - C - C = C - C - C - C - C - C - C - O - H
    |   |           |   |   |   |   |
    H   H           H   H   H   H   H
```

Fig. 3.1

For our purposes, the three key omega-3 fatty acids are:

- alpha linolenic acid (ALA)
- eicosapentaenoic acid (EPA)
- docosahexaenoic acid (DHA)

Through the 1980s and 1990s, several randomized, controlled studies published in the *New England Journal of Medicine* and other prestigious medical journals suggested that omega-3 fatty acids could lower blood pressure.[13] Meanwhile, researchers looking at the diets and overall health of large groups of people found that small amounts of fish might lower the risk of coronary heart disease[14] and result in less arrhythmias and sudden death problems linked to hypertension.

We haven't yet identified all the ways in which the omega-3s reduce blood pressure and lower the risk of associated diseases, but we do know that ALA snatches away certain enzymes the body might otherwise use to produce substances that prompt inflammation and the thickening of the blood. The omega-3s, in general, spur the body to increase production of substances that encourage the blood vessels to relax, thus reducing blood pressure. Omega-3s also help improve insulin sensitivity and enhance the action of specific cell walls (membranes). Through these and possibly other mechanisms, the omega-3s help:

- reduce blood pressure
- quell inflammation
- reduce the tendency of platelets to stick together unnecessarily
- reduce fibrinogen (a blood-clotting protein)
- reduce irregular heartbeat (arrhythmia)
- reduce blood fat
- reduce atherosclerosis, coronary heart disease, and heart attack

The protective effect of omega-3s has been documented in study after study. For example:

• A 1989 study published in the *New England Journal of Medicine*[15] reported that blood pressure dropped significantly in fifteen hypertensive subjects given 15 grams of fish oil per day.

- Ten years after that, a study appearing in the *American Journal of Clinical Nutrition*[16] looked at sixty-three people with hypertension and hyperlipidemia (elevated cholesterol and blood fats). After taking 3.65 grams of omega-3 fatty acids for sixteen weeks, their blood pressure levels fell significantly.
- A study of 399 healthy males showed that increasing the amount of ALA in fatty tissue by only 1 percent was associated with a 5 mm Hg drop in the systolic and diastolic blood pressure.[17]

A paper published in *Circulation*[18] gave an overview of the situation by combining the results of thirty-one different fish oil–hypertension studies. The authors of this study concluded that fish oil does indeed reduce blood pressure in people with mild hypertension, and the larger the dose, the better the results:

- Less than 4 grams of fish oil per day = no change in blood pressure
- Between 4 and 7 grams per day = a drop of 1.6 to 2.9 mm Hg
- More than 15 grams per day = a drop of 5.8 to 8.1 mm Hg

But the omega-3s are smart. They don't fix it if it's not broken, which means that normal blood pressure remains normal.

Another study, published in the journal *Hypertension*,[19] looked at what happened when hypertensive, overweight people were asked to take fish oil *and* lose weight. Sixty-three overweight and hypertensive men and women, ranging in age from forty to seventy, were enlisted in the study. Their systolic blood pressures were between 125 and 180, while their diastolic pressures were as high as 109. Everybody was asked to cut back on salt intake. Then the volunteers were divided into groups. Group 1 made no changes in their diet or weight. Group 2 ate one fish meal a day. Group 3 lost weight. Group 4 ate one fish meal per day *and* lost weight. Here's what happened:

- Those who ate one fish meal a day decreased their systolic BP by 6.0 mm Hg and diastolic BP by 3.0 mm Hg.
- Those who lost weight decreased their systolic BP by 5.5 mm Hg and diastolic BP by 2.2 mm Hg.
- Those who ate a fish meal *and* lost weight decreased their systolic BP by 13.0 mm Hg and diastolic BP by 9.3 mm Hg.

The researchers reported that "the effects were large," and concluded that when fish was added to the diet and people lost weight, their risk of cardiovascular disease and need for antihypertensive drugs were likely to decrease substantially. I was particularly struck by this study, for it highlights the point that there is no single best way to combat hypertension. It must be attacked on several fronts at once.

I recommend an intake of 3 to 4 grams of omega-3 fatty acids per day. Eating cold-water fish such as herring, mackerel, and salmon daily is as effective as taking omega-3 supplements such as EPA and DHA.

There's still a lot more to learn about the omega-3 fatty acids. For example, it appears that DHA has a stronger effect on blood pressure than does than EPA, and that EPA is stronger than ALA. We'll undoubtedly fine-tune our recommendations as we learn more, but for now it's quite clear that the omega-3 fatty acids can be powerful tools in the fight against hypertension.

A FEW WORDS ON OMEGA-6S

Although the omega-6 fatty acids don't usually lower blood pressure significantly, they do have properties that make them useful in the battle against elevated blood pressure. They can help protect against increases in blood pressure caused by saturated fats, enhance the manufacture of substances that relax the arteries, block stress-induced hypertension, and otherwise help the pressure remain on an even keel. GLA (gamma linolenic acid) is perhaps the best known of the omega-6s. You'll find omega-6 fatty acids in sesame seed oil and seeds, unrefined corn oil, canola oil, nuts, evening primrose oil, borage seed oil, and black currant oil. I recommend an intake of 2 to 4 grams of flaxseed oil daily or a GLA supplement, 240 mg twice a day.

OLIVE OIL

For years, researchers have been intrigued by the fact that people living in Greece, Italy, and surrounding countries who consume the Mediterranean diet have fewer problems with hypertension and heart disease than we who consume the standard Western diet. One of the differences between the two diets is the olive oil that's used in many Mediterranean recipes. Olive oil is rich in monounsaturated fatty acids (MUFAs) such as the omega-9 fatty acid called *oleic acid*, and contains some polyunsaturated fatty acids as well. The studies on MUFAs, in general, and olive oil, in particular, have been impressive:

• A study appearing in the *Archives of Internal Medicine*[20] in the year 2000 described what happened when twenty-three people suffering from hypertension were given either extra virgin olive oil or sunflower oil. (Sunflower oil is a typical oil used in standard Western diets.) This was a six-month, double-blind, randomized study. (*Double-blind* means that neither the researchers nor the volunteers knew who was receiving what until the end of the study period. *Randomized* means that the volunteers were randomly assigned to receive either the olive or sunflower oil.) Compared to sunflower oil, olive oil decreased systolic blood pressure an additional 8 mm Hg and diastolic pressure an additional 6 mm Hg. Not only that, the need for antihypertensive medications was reduced by 48 percent in the olive oil group, compared to only 4 percent in the sunflower group.

- In another study,[21] the systolic and diastolic blood pressure rose when olive oil was removed from the Mediterranean diet the test subjects were eating, and replaced with the saturated fatty acids so common in the standard Western diet.

As with the omega-3 fatty acids, it's still up in the air as to why olive oil has such a beneficial effect on hypertension. We do know that, among other things, MUFAs make nitric oxide more bioavailable, which makes it better able to keep the arteries dilated, help combat the ill effects of oxidation, and improve endothelial function.

I recommend an intake of MUFAs in the form of 4 tablespoons of extra virgin olive oil per day.

VITAMIN C

Vitamin C leapt into the public eye in the 1970s when Dr. Linus Pauling and others announced that it could reduce the severity of the common cold. Through the years we've learned that vitamin C plays an important role in regulating blood pressure and decreasing it in hypertensives.

We know from population, observational, and experimental

studies that the amount of vitamin C in the diet and/or in the blood plasma is inversely related to the systolic and diastolic blood pressure, as well as to the heart rate.[22] That is, the more C in the diet and/or blood plasma, the lower the two pressures and the heart rate. The NHANES-II study (National Health and Nutrition Examination Survey, a long-range study that has been following some 14,000 Americans since 1975) found low levels of plasma vitamin C in 20 percent of white men and 30 percent of black men. The fact that blacks are more likely than whites to have lower blood levels of vitamin C may partially explain why a greater percentage of African-Americans develop hypertension.

We've also learned that the greater the quantity of vitamin C consumed, the lower the risk of cardiovascular disease, coronary heart disease, and stroke. There are many studies on vitamin C and blood pressure. Let's take a brief look at just a few of them:

- Twenty-three hypertensive women were followed for three months. Their blood pressures ranged from 149/90 to 160/100. Taking 1 gram (1,000 mg) of vitamin C per day reduced the average systolic pressure by 7 mm Hg, and the average diastolic pressure by 4 mm Hg.[23]

- Twelve people with hypertension were given 1 gram of vitamin C orally every day for six weeks in a randomized, crossover study. Their average systolic blood pressure fell by 5 mm Hg, their average diastolic by 1 mm Hg.[24]

- Thirty-nine hypertensives with diastolic blood pressures ranging from 90 to 110 mm Hg were enrolled in a placebo-controlled, four-week study. After an initial loading dose of 2,000 mg of vitamin C, the participants were given 500 mg of C per day. Their systolic blood pressures fell an average of 11 mm Hg, their diastolic an average of 6 mm Hg.[25]

- A very interesting study[26] was reported in the *Journal of Hypertension* in 2000. This was a six-month-long, double-blind, randomized, placebo-controlled, crossover study. The forty men and women in the study, ranging in age from sixty to eighty, had mild hypertension or no hypertension at all. For three months they were given either 250 mg of vitamin C twice daily, or a placebo. Then they took nothing for a week, before switching. (Those taking the C then took the placebo; and those on the placebo now took the C.) At first glance, the results were moderate, showing a decrease in systolic, but not the diastolic, pressure. But then the researchers noted that the higher the participant's blood pressure had been at the start, the greater their response to the vitamin C. So the researchers tallied the results again, this time looking only at those with hypertension. The reduction in pressure was now more pronounced and significant, and they concluded that vitamin C reduces the daytime systolic blood pressure in those with hypertension, but not in people with normal blood pressure.

To date, we've identified several ways in which vitamin C works. The vitamin improves endothelial dysfunction in people with hypertension. In patients with coronary heart disease, it restores arteries to their relaxed state. Giving vitamin C, whether orally or intravenously, reverses endothelial dysfunction and causes the arteries to dilate in those with coronary heart disease and in smokers.

This much is clear from numerous studies: Blood pressure is inversely correlated with vitamin C intake and the amount of C in the blood plasma. Taking vitamin C reduces the blood pressure in those with hypertension, hyperlipidemia, and diabetes, or combinations of these diseases. The higher the blood pressure is to begin with, the more it falls. And combining vitamin

C with other antioxidants, such as vitamin E, beta-carotene, or selenium, enhances its ability to reduce hypertension.

> ### C FACTS
>
> Although they had no idea what vitamin C was, ancient mariners knew what happened when you didn't get enough of it. Many a sailor on a long voyage, unable to eat the fresh fruits and vegetables that contain vitamin C, developed inflamed and swollen joints, rotting and bleeding gums, slow wound healing, weakness, fatigue, depression, and hysteria. Today we know that these are the signs of scurvy, a deadly disease that was the scourge of the high seas.
>
> *Duties:* We need vitamin C to keep the immune system strong; manufacture and maintain the collagen in our bones, skin, blood vessels, and elsewhere in the body; and to fight off certain types of cancer; among other things.
>
> *Deficiency:* A severe deficiency of C can cause scurvy. More typically we see mild deficiencies that cause muscle cramps, slow wound healing, and inflammation of the gums.
>
> *Excess:* Excessive dosages (over 2 grams per day) can cause diarrhea.

I recommend an intake of 250 to 500 mg of vitamin C twice a day in supplement form. You can also find vitamin C in papayas, guavas, red peppers, cantaloupes, black currants, green peppers, oranges, broccoli, cauliflower, and asparagus.

COENZYME Q_{10}

When researchers first discovered coenzyme Q_{10} (or CoQ_{10}, for short), they named it *ubiquinone* because it was found everywhere (ubiquitous) in the body and it belonged to the quinone family of compounds. The word *coenzyme* means an enzyme that works with other enzymes to keep the body's metabolic machinery humming along efficiently. Although it's vital to life, it's not considered an essential nutrient because we can manufacture it in our bodies. We also take in small amounts of CoQ_{10} when we eat meat and seafood.

Widely used in Europe and Japan, CoQ_{10} is an ingredient in over 200 different Japanese preparations,[27] and is given to millions of people suffering from cardiovascular disease.[28] In this country, Europe, and Japan, CoQ_{10} has been studied extensively and is used to treat congestive heart failure, angina, hypertension, and other ailments.

CoQ_{10} has many functions in the body. It improves the action of the mitochondria, the tiny energy factories inside the cell. It acts as a powerful antioxidant, and helps to keep the total cholesterol down. We manufacture—or should be able to manufacture—all of the CoQ_{10} we need but, unfortunately, our blood levels of CoQ_{10} decrease with age. They're also lower in people with hypertension, atherosclerosis, diabetes mellitus, and other diseases in which oxidation is a problem, and in those taking statin (anticholesterol) drugs.

There's a strong link between CoQ_{10} and hypertension, which can be summed up as follows:

- People with essential hypertension are more likely to have a CoQ_{10} deficiency than those without hypertension (39 percent compared to 6 percent).
- In studies involving hypertensive patients, oral adminis-

tration of 100 to 225 mg of CoQ_{10} per day triggers a significant and consistent reduction in blood pressure.[29]

In these studies, the systolic blood pressure falls by an average of 15 mm Hg, and the diastolic by 10 mm Hg.

• Those who begin the study with the lowest levels of serum CoQ_{10} seem to respond the best when given supplemental CoQ_{10}.

• CoQ_{10} is not fast-acting; it takes about four weeks for it to reach its peak effect. And about two weeks after you stop using it, blood pressure will return to its original levels.

• CoQ_{10} is often powerful enough to allow patients to reduce or eliminate their hypertensive drugs. Approximately 50 percent of patients taking antihypertensive medications may be able to stop taking one to three of them. (Many hypertensives are on multiple medications.)

• CoQ_{10} is remarkably well tolerated. Even at high doses, it does not trigger any serious or chronic adverse effects.

CoQ_{10} also improves some of the risk factors for cardiovascular disease. Among other things, it reduces total cholesterol and LDL ("bad") cholesterol, improves carbohydrate metabolism and insulin sensitivity, lowers blood glucose, reduces oxidative stress, decreases the heart rate, improves oxygen delivery, and may improve heart function.

I recommend an intake of 60 to 120 mg of CoQ_{10} in supplement form, once a day or in divided doses. Be sure, however, that your supplement is certified, bioavailable, of the highest quality, and that it contains a consistent amount of CoQ_{10}.

This is very important, as clinical trials have shown that all brands of CoQ_{10} are *not* equivalent. I recommend to my patients that they use any brand that utilizes a patented form of

CoQ_{10} known as Q-Gel®. Q-Gel® is a newer, solubilized form of CoQ_{10} that is more bioavailable, which means that more of it is available for the body to use.

In 1998, the *International Journal for Vitamin and Nutrition Research* published a study that compared, in humans, the relative bioavailability of Q-Gel® to that of typical commercially available forms of CoQ_{10}. Standard softgel capsules, hardshell capsules, and powder-based tablets were all tested against Q-Gel® using a daily dosage of 120 mg per day for three weeks. The baseline plasma CoQ_{10} values were all very comparable prior to the study (0.50–0.52 mg/mL). After three weeks the values were 1.37, 1.63, and 1.60 mg/mL for the softgels, capsules, and tablets—but were much higher for Q-Gel® at 3.31 mg/mL. This is key, for you need this higher level in the blood in order to fight the diseases we've been discussing.

The results from this initial study were replicated in a second study, allowing us to say that Q-Gel® is vastly superior to typical CoQ_{10} preparations. This means a savings for consumers, for you can take lower doses of Q-Gel® yet still rapidly reach and maintain good blood levels of CoQ_{10}. When you're looking for CoQ_{10} in pharmacies and health food stores, I advise you, like I do my patients: Select a product that uses the form of CoQ_{10} known as Q-Gel®.

For a list of CoQ_{10} brands that use Q-Gel®, please go to www.tishcon.com. On the home page, look for and click on the link to Q-Gel®, then click on "Ordering Information" to get a list of companies that use Q-Gel® in their CoQ_{10} product.

VITAMIN E

Vitamin E's ability to lower blood pressure has been studied extensively in animals, but only a few studies have been performed on humans suffering from hypertension. If the vitamin does work directly to lower blood pressure, its effect is probably small and may be limited to those who have hypertension *plus* vascular disease, diabetes, or other problems.

Still, there's a clear link between E and hypertension. Studies show us that hypertensive patients have significantly lower levels of E in their plasma and cells as compared to normotensives (those with normal blood pressure levels). Why? It's probably due to vitamin E's ability to improve endothelial function, thus reducing the damage to the vascular system and other organs that are typically harmed by elevated blood pressure. And, of course, the vitamin is also a powerful antioxidant. Because it's fat-soluble, it can insert itself into cell membranes (which are made up of fatty substances), where it helps stop free radical chain reactions that can damage or kill otherwise healthy cells.

E FACTS

Believe it or not, there are *eight* different forms of vitamin E. Or perhaps it's better to say that there are eight naturally occurring compounds that demonstrate characteristic vitamin E biological activity.

Four of these substances are *tocopherols* (alpha-tocopherol, beta-tocopherol, gamma-tocopherol, delta-tocopherol) and four are *tocotrienols* (alpha-tocotrienol, beta-tocotrienol, gamma-tocotrienol, and delta-tocotrienol). Alpha-tocopherol has long been thought to be the most biologically active form of E, the one with the most E-ness. But that belief appears to be changing as new studies delve into the prowess of the four

> tocotrienols. For the sake of convenience, we will refer to the eight forms collectively as vitamin E.
>
> *Duties:* Vitamin E protects the muscles, eyes, skin, and other parts of the body from oxidative damage, guards against damage to the red blood cells, and wards off pollution-induced damage to the lungs and mouth.
>
> *Deficiency:* A deficiency of vitamin E can lead to premature aging of the skin, infertility, destruction of red blood cells, and nervous system disorders.
>
> *Excess:* Large doses of vitamin E can interfere with vitamin K's role in the clotting of the blood, causing excessive bleeding. This is especially dangerous if megadoses of vitamin E are taken in conjunction with blood-thinning medications. Generally, a dosage of 400 to 800 IU of vitamin E is considered safe.

I recommend an intake of 400 to 800 IU of mixed natural vitamin E daily in supplement form. The supplement should contain all four tocopherols and all four tocotrienols. You can also find vitamin E in leafy green vegetables, whole grains, wheat germ, nuts, liver, butter, and egg yolk.

FLAVONOIDS

Flavonoids are a large group of natural substances found in fruits, vegetables, grains, tea, wine, and licorice. So far, over 4,000 different flavonoids have been identified, including the rutin found in cranberries, the epicatechin in green tea, and the quercetin in red wine, olives, onions, parsley, and lettuce.

Several major studies have shown that the flavonoids are powerful free radical scavengers with antihypertensive properties. These studies also show that they prevent atherosclerosis and promote the relaxation of muscles surrounding the arteries, allowing the arteries to dilate. Flavonoids such as daidzein and genistein, which are both found in soy, lower total cholesterol and LDL ("bad") cholesterol, while reducing the formation of blood clots in the coronary arteries and elsewhere. The quercetin in red wine reduces oxidation of LDL and the tendency of platelets to stick together unnecessarily. The catechins in green tea can help relax the muscles around the arteries, lower cholesterol, prevent oxidation of LDL, and keep platelets from clumping together unnecessarily.

In a recent study,[30] researchers tested the effects of the *Achillea wilhelmsii*, a plant that's rich in flavonoids, in 120 men and women suffering from high blood pressure and elevated cholesterol. Over a six-month period, the plant significantly lowered both the systolic and diastolic blood pressures. It also reduced the total cholesterol, LDL, and blood fats, while pushing up the level of the HDL ("good") cholesterol.

Although we need more studies, it's clear that the flavonoids are helpful in the fight against hypertension. Many of the flavonoids relax the vascular musculature, thus reducing the resistance portion of the blood pressure equation. They reduce total cholesterol and LDL ("bad") cholesterol, and deactivate dangerous free radicals. They also have anti-inflammatory effects,[31] which means they can help reduce the number of arterial scratches that lead to atherosclerosis. And consider this: The flavonoids are found in delicious foods like apples, cherries, grapes, lettuce, onions, parsley, raspberries, strawberries, citrus fruits, broccoli, celery, and green tea. All of these foods are part of the DASH-I and DASH-II diets, the major diets proven to reduce blood pressure. So even if the flavonoids by themselves don't reduce your blood pressure to healthy levels, they're part of the overall answer. And they're appealing to both the eye and the palate.

I recommend eating several servings of flavonoid-containing foods daily.

VITAMIN B_6

The fact that vitamin B_6 plays a role in keeping blood pressure normal isn't surprising, as this vitamin affects many parts of the body. Studies have shown that low levels of B_6 in the blood serum are linked to hypertension,[32] and that giving supplemental B_6 to hypertensive animals reduces their blood pressure. In a study with humans,[33] researchers compared nine normotensive men and women to twenty people with hypertension. Taking supplemental B_6 for four weeks caused the systolic pressure to fall 8.5 percent, and the diastolic to fall 9.3 percent.

Vitamin B_6 has multiple antihypertensive effects that resemble those of diuretics, calcium channel blockers, and central alpha agonists, some of the major medicines for hypertension.

B_6 FACTS

Vitamin B_6, also known as pyridoxine, is part of the B family of vitamins. In a sense, vitamin B_6 itself is a sub-family, since it consists of three different compounds.

Duties: Vitamin B_6 helps the body extract energy from carbohydrates, proteins, and fats. It's also necessary for the production of hemoglobin, neurotransmitters, and hormones, and helps convert amino acids into carbohydrates. The vitamin may also help relieve the symptoms of premenstrual syndrome, carpal tunnel syndrome, and certain mood disorders. Particularly important is the ability of vitamin B_6 to recycle the compound homocysteine by turning it into the amino acid methionine. A buildup of homocysteine in the blood is believed to damage the endothelium and bring on atherosclerosis.

Deficiency: A lack of B_6 can trigger a host of rather vague symptoms, including lowered immunity, loss of appetite, insomnia, lethargy, and irregular heartbeat.

Excess: Dosages up to 200 mg per day are safe and typically have no adverse effects. However, long-term dosages of 500 mg per day can lead to irreversible nerve damage.

I recommend an intake of 100 to 200 mg of vitamin B_6 every day, the bulk of it from food. You can also find vitamin B_6 in avocados, beef liver, bananas, chicken, smoked salmon, red snapper, wheat germ, corn, and yogurt.

ZINC

Studies have found that low blood levels of zinc are associated with hypertension, coronary artery disease, Type II diabetes, elevated blood fats, lowered HDL ("good") cholesterol, and possibly insulin resistance.[34] Zinc's antihypertensive effects may be due to its ability to inhibit the expression of unfavorable genes, reduce insulin resistance, inhibit the body's blood-pressure-elevating system (the renin-angiotensin-aldosterone system), and slow the increase in blood pressure prompted by the stimulation of the sympathetic nervous system.

> ## Zinc Facts
>
> Although we've known since the early 1900s that farm animals need zinc, we didn't realize it was an essential nutrient for humans until the 1970s.
>
> *Duties:* Zinc helps to keep the memory intact and the immune system strong, aids in reproduction, keeps the blood sugar at normal levels, and is necessary for strong bones.
>
> *Deficiency:* A lack of zinc can lead to anorexia, delayed sexual maturity, fatigue, diarrhea, impotency, increased infections, poor vision, irritability, memory difficulties, paranoia, and slow wound healing.
>
> *Excess:* Too much zinc can interfere with copper metabolism, and in some cases can reduce the heart-protective HDL ("good") cholesterol by as much as 15 percent. Excess intake of zinc can result in diarrhea, nausea, cramps, vomiting, and a lowered immunity.

I recommend an intake of 25 mg of zinc per day in supplement form. You can also find zinc in oysters, calf's liver, wheat germ, sardines, yogurt, and eggs.

CELERY

Back in the nineteenth century, celery was considered a delicacy—an exotic and expensive vegetable to be served only at fancy dinners in specially designed celery dishes. You could actually purchase celery gum and celery soda, and the Sears & Roebuck catalogue sold a celery elixir as a treatment for nervous ailments. Although celery's popularity plummeted when it became cheap enough for everyone to afford, recent findings about its health benefits are liable to make it much more interesting.

In studies with animals, a component of celery oil called 3-n-butyl phthalide reduced blood pressure significantly. In a Chinese study, blood pressure fell significantly in fourteen of sixteen hypertensives who were given celery.

We don't know all the ways celery helps us, but we do know that it contains a substance called *apigenin*, which, among other things, helps lower blood pressure. Celery also acts like a diuretic or ACE 1, helping rid the body of excess fluid, which may be one way it reduces elevated blood pressure.

I recommend the following intake of celery: Either 4 celery stalks per day, 8 teaspoons of celery juice 3 times daily, 1,000 mg of celery seed extract twice a day, or ½ to 1 teaspoon of celery oil 3 times daily in tincture form.

GARLIC AND ALLICIN

A very popular herbal supplement, with sales second only to echinacea, garlic has been used as a health aid for a very long time. Workers in ancient Egypt used garlic to enhance their strength, Greek soldiers to heal wounds, and seventeenth-century English physicians to treat smallpox. More recently, garlic has gained recognition for its ability to relieve hypertension. Several clinical trials have consistently shown that the correct type and dose of garlic reduces blood pressure in hypertensives,[35] resulting in a typical fall in systolic pressure of between 5 and 8 mm Hg.[36]

Garlic contains several substances that may account for its ability to lower elevated blood pressure, including natural ACE inhibitors (such as gamma-glutamyl peptides and flavonolic compounds), magnesium (which relaxes the arterial muscle and is a natural calcium channel blocker), ajoenes, phosphorus, adenosine, allicin, and sulfur compounds. These and other compounds in garlic allow it to help the body keep the arteries dilated, thus reducing vascular resistance and blood pressure.

I recommend an intake of 4 cloves or 4 grams of garlic daily.

Caution: All garlic preparations are *not* processed in the same way, and they do *not* have the same potency. In addition, cultivated garlic (*Allium sativum*), wild uncultivated garlic or bear garlic (*Allium urisinum*), and aged or fresh garlic will have variable effects, depending on growing conditions, the way the garlic has been transported and stored, and so forth. I've had success using Kyolic Aged Garlic Extract™.

SEAWEED

Seaweed can do more than just hold your sushi rolls together; it's also a powerful aid in the battle against blood pressure. In a study[37] with animals, wakame seaweed inhibited the clamping down of the tiny muscles surrounding the arteries and reduced blood pressure as well as captopril, one of the standard drugs for hypertension. In a study with humans, taking 3.3 grams of dried wakame for four weeks reduced the systolic blood pressure by 14 mm Hg, and significantly lowered the diastolic pressure as well.[38] Another study[39] looked at sixty-two middle-aged men with mild hypertension. Giving the men 12 or 24 grams of a special seaweed preparation for four weeks caused the blood pressure to fall by an average of 11.2 mm Hg in the sodium-sensitive subjects, and 5.7 mm Hg in the non-sodium-sensitive subjects.

Wakame seaweed appears to ease hypertension through its

inhibiting effect on the muscles that constrict blood vessels. In other words, it's a natural ACE inhibitor. Other varieties of seaweed may help reduce blood pressure by increasing the intestinal absorption of potassium while reducing the absorption of sodium.

I recommend an intake of 3.0 to 3.5 grams (2 tablespoons) of dried wakame seaweed per day.

FIBER

Fiber has been praised for its ability to lower cholesterol and improve bowel function. Different sources of fiber—guar gum, guava, psyllium, and oat bran—can also reduce blood pressure and the need for medication in hypertensives, as well as in diabetics and in patients with both diseases.[40]

Fiber fights hypertension and its ill effects by reducing endothelial dysfunction, encouraging the body to excrete sodium via the urine, improving insulin sensitivity, and decreasing the sympathetic nervous system activity that can increase blood pressure.

Two recent studies[41] have reported a decrease in systolic pressure of 7.5 to 9.4 mm Hg and 5.5 mm Hg in diastolic pressure in hypertensives given different forms of fiber (glucomannan in one study, oat bran in the other). In addition, both soluble and insoluble fiber can reduce total cholesterol, LDL ("bad") cholesterol, and blood fats, while increasing the HDL ("good") cholesterol.

In order to see drops of this magnitude, I recommend a daily intake of one of the following: 60 grams (2.1 ounces) of oatmeal, 40 grams (1.4 ounces) of oat bran, 3 grams (0.25 ounce) of beta-glucan (a type of fiber), or 7 grams (0.1 ounce) of psyllium.

L-ARGININE

L-arginine is a specific form of the amino acid arginine, one of the many building blocks of protein. L-arginine is used by the body to make nitric oxide, which helps to reduce constriction of the blood vessels, improve endothelial dysfunction, and lower the blood pressure.

Giving L-arginine intravenously to salt-sensitive hypertensives can help reduce blood pressure. L-arginine also has medicinal effects on coronary disease. Giving patients 10 grams per day increases blood flow through the coronary arteries and elsewhere in the body, decreases the pain of angina, and reduces the symptoms of peripheral vascular disease.

L-arginine produces a biologically significant decrease in blood pressure, almost equal to the results you can expect when consuming the DASH-I diet.[42] It does this at doses of 10 grams per day, whether in food or supplement form.[43] This dose of L-arginine appears to be safe, but long-term human studies supporting this have yet to be published.

I recommend an intake of 5 grams of L-arginine twice daily in supplement form or foods: You can find arginine in lentils, hazelnuts, walnuts, and peanuts.

HAWTHORN BERRY

Hawthorn berry is an herb that was used by the ancients to treat sleep and digestive problems. Modern studies indicate that it may also lower blood pressure and cholesterol, dilate the coronary arteries, reduce the incidence of irregular heartbeat, and otherwise combat hypertension, cardiovascular disease, and related ailments.

Hawthorn berry is an ACE inhibitor; that is, it works by inhibiting the angiotensin-converting enzyme that would otherwise cause constriction of the arteries. Hawthorn berry also contains various flavonoids, which have effects similar to beta blockers, calcium channel blockers, and diuretics. It contains rutin, magnesium, chromium, catechin, and several other phytochemicals, all of which may work to combat high blood pressure.

I recommend a daily intake of 160 to 900 mg of standardized hawthorn extract.

TAURINE

Taurine is an amino acid that the body *doesn't* use to make protein. Instead, it circulates freely throughout the brain, retina, and heart muscle. Studies have shown that taurine can lower both blood pressure and heart rate, while decreasing irregular heart rhythms and the symptoms of congestive heart failure. In a study of nineteen people with hypertension, giving 6 grams of taurine per day for 7 days reduced the systolic blood pressure by 9 mm Hg and the diastolic by 4.1 mm Hg.[44]

I recommend an intake of 1.0 to 1.5 grams of taurine twice a day in supplement form.

L-CARNITINE

L-carnitine is a nitrogen-based substance that helps the body oxidize fatty acids. Although there are only limited human studies involving L-carnitine, the clinical and experimental trials have shown that it's useful in treating hypertension, diabetes mellitus, ischemic heart disease, claudication, acute heart attack, congestive heart failure, irregular heartbeat, elevated cholesterol and/or blood fats, and other ailments.

I recommend an intake of 1,000 mg of L-carnitine twice a day in supplement form (taken early in the day).

N-ACETYL CYSTEINE

N-acetyl cysteine, a form of the amino acid cysteine, is a powerful antioxidant that can improve endothelial function in the aorta, that giant artery that rises up out of the heart. It increases nitric oxide levels, relaxing the muscles surrounding the arteries. This, in turn, lowers homocysteine, increases glutathionine, reduces arterial resistance and lowers blood pressure.

N-acetyl cysteine is a natural calcium channel blocker, which makes it useful in treating hypertension. It also reverses platelet aggregation and has other beneficial effects on the blood vessels.

I recommend an intake of 500 mg of n-acetyl cysteine twice a day in supplement form.

ALPHA LIPOIC ACID (Lipoic Acid or Thioctic Acid)

Alpha lipoic acid is a powerful antioxidant that can pinch-hit for other antioxidants, such as vitamins C or E, when you run short of them. So far, the only studies on alpha lipoic acid and hypertension have been performed on animals. The results have been impressive, with alpha lipoic acid driving down the systolic blood pressure, and possibly even reducing the damage to the arteries caused by the incessant flow of blood.

Alpha lipoic acid improves endothelial dysfunction and hinders the action of the white blood cells, which bind to the endothelium wherever there is a scratch and trigger the development of atherosclerosis. It's also a natural calcium channel blocker.

I recommend an intake of 100 to 200 mg of alpha lipoic acid twice a day in supplement form. Since taking alpha lipoic acid can increase your need for biotin, I also recommend 800 mcg of biotin twice a day. Biotin, a member of the B family of vitamins, has several functions in the body, including the aiding of the conversion of blood glucose into energy.

LYCOPENE

Lycopene, a cousin to beta-carotene and a powerful antioxidant, can significantly reduce blood pressure, according to studies presented in 2001.[45] One of these studies[46] looked at thirty people, ages forty to sixty-five, suffering from stage 1 hypertension. After taking a lycopene extract for eight weeks, their average systolic blood pressure fell from 144 to 135 mm Hg, and their diastolic from 91 to 84 mm Hg, very significant results.

I recommend an intake of 10 mg of lycopene per day in supplement form. You can also find lycopene in tomatoes and tomato products, guavas, pink grapefruit, watermelons, apricots, papayas, red peppers, and strawberries.

GUAVA FRUIT

A study in the *Journal of Human Hypertension*[47] pointed out some interesting possibilities involving this tasty fruit. Seventy-two people with essential hypertension were given 0.5 to 1.0 gram of guava fruit daily (the equivalent of one to two medium guavas) in a randomized, single-blind, placebo-controlled study. (Single-blind means that the participants didn't know if they were getting the real thing or the placebo during the course of the study, although the researchers knew.)

Four weeks later, those who ate the guava had an average drop of 7.5 mm Hg in systolic BP and 8.5 mm Hg in diastolic BP. The large amount of soluble fiber, vitamin C, potassium, and other nutrients in the guava may be responsible for its beneficial effects.

HERBS

Through the years, various herbs have been put forth as treatments for hypertension. Unfortunately, the studies supporting most of them have been small or inconclusive. While that doesn't mean that some herbs won't prove worthwhile, it does mean that we can't make any definitive statements yet.

The herbs that some experts believe are beneficial for easing hypertension include ashwagandha, jiaogulan, onions and onion oil, maitake mushrooms, dill, lemon or lemon peel, purslane, yinyanghuo, devil's claw, kudzu root or tea, guar gum, kaffir potato, reishi, skullcap, Siberian ginseng, capsicum, fumitory, ginger, angelica, anise, banana, baytree, cashew, echinacea, eucalyptus, German chamomile, ginkgo biloba, Indian mulberry, lotus, neem, nutmeg, puncture vine, and St. John's wort.

WHEW!

We've talked about a lot of substances in this chapter, everything from alpha linolenic acid to zinc. It may feel overwhelming, impossible to master. But don't worry. In the next chapter you'll find the short list of helpful supplements. If you just take those, you're making a great start. And in Chapter 5 you'll learn about the ideal diet for lowering blood pressure. Switching from the typical American fast food diet to this health-enhancing way of eating will give you more of many of the substances we discussed in this chapter.

If you can jump right into the deep end and adopt the helpful recommendations in this book all at once, great. If not, start by dipping your toe in the shallow end, and move on from there.

MIMICKING THE MEDICINES

The foods and food substances we talked about in this chapter can behave much like the medicines that doctors prescribe for hypertension. Here are some lists of foods and supplements that can have medicine-like actions.

Foods and Supplements That Can Act As Diuretics

Hawthorn berry	GLA	Calcium (Ca^{++})
Vitamin B$_6$	Vitamin C	Protein
Taurine	Potassium (K$^+$)	Fiber
Celery	Magnesium (Mg^{++})	Coenzyme Q$_{10}$

Foods and Supplements That Can Act As Central Alpha Agonists

Taurine	Sodium restriction	Vitamin C
Potassium (K$^+$)	Protein	Vitamin B$_6$
Zinc	Fiber	Coenzyme Q$_{10}$
Celery	GLA/DGLA	Garlic

Foods and Supplements That Can Act As Direct Vasodilators

Omega-3 fatty acids	Fiber	L-arginine
MUFAs (omega-9s)	Garlic	Taurine
Potassium (K$^+$)	Flavonoids	Celery

The Multifaceted Solution

Magnesium (MG^{++})	Vitamin C	Alpha lipoic acid
Calcium (Ca^{++})	Vitamin E	
Soy	Coenzyme Q$_{10}$	

Foods and Supplements That Can Act As Calcium Channel Blockers

Alpha lipoic acid	Hawthorn berry
Vitamin C	Celery
Vitamin B$_6$	Omega-3 fatty acids (EPA and DHA)
Magnesium (Mg^{++})	Calcium
N-acetyl cysteine	Garlic
Vitamin E	

Foods and Supplements That Can Act As Angiotensin-Converting Enzyme Inhibitors (ACEIs)

Garlic	Gelatin
Seaweed	Sake
Tuna protein/muscle	Omega-3 fatty acids
Sardine protein/muscle	Chicken egg yolks
Hawthorn berry	Zein
Bonito fish (dried)	Dried salted fish
Pycnogenol	Fish sauce
Casein	Zinc
Hydrolyzed whey protein	Hydrolyzed wheat germ isolate
Sour milk	

Foods and Supplements That Can Act As Angiotensin II Receptor Blockers (ARBs)

Potassium	Vitamin B_6
Fiber	CoQ_{10}
Garlic	Celery
Vitamin C	GLA and DGLA

Foods and Supplements That Can Act As Beta Blockers

Hawthorn berry

Chapter 4

The *Hypertension Institute Program*

In a perfect world, I'd be able to recommend a couple of all-natural supplements that you'd take with your orange juice at breakfast and, magically, your blood pressure would settle down into the normal range and stay there for good. But in the real world, nothing is quite that easy. Although we've seen how numerous foods and supplements can do much to ease your hypertension, the best results occur when they are part of a larger program. That's why I've developed the *Hypertension Institute Program*, the ten-step program that I recommend to patients at my clinic. It's based on the best parts of both conventional and alternative medicine.

Step 1: See Your Physician Regularly

If you have hypertension, it is absolutely vital that you see your doctor regularly. Blood pressure may move up or down over time, especially if you're suffering from an underlying condition like atherosclerosis that makes things worse. And then there are the various lifestyle issues that can drive your pressure up, including weight gain, lack of exercise, excessive stress, a high intake of alcohol, and smoking. Since there are so many variables involved and your blood pressure can rise at any time, you *must* have it checked—and checked often—by your physician. But a more likely outcome, after reading this book and applying its principles, is that you'll go to your physician and hear the good news: Your blood pressure is coming down.

But before beginning this program, schedule an appointment with your doctor. Let him or her know what you'd like to do, just in case there's any reason why another approach may be best for you.

THE RIGHT WAY TO MEASURE BP

It seems like it should be a no-brainer: Dash into the doc's office, plop down in the seat. The doctor or nurse wraps the cuff around your arm, pumps it up with air, puts the stethoscope on your arm, deflates the cuff, listens for some sounds, then marks down the numbers. Easy, right? Wrong.

The procedure is far more complex, which means that carelessness can lead to an improper reading. Ideally, you should be sitting down for a full five minutes before the cuff is applied. The room in which you're sitting should be quiet, the chair comfortable. You should not have had any food or caffeine, and should not have smoked, exerted yourself, or been exposed to extreme temperatures for at least an hour.

The cuff should be an appropriate size for your arm. This means that the cuff bladder, the part that inflates, should be

20 percent wider than the diameter of your arm, and about twice as long as it is wide. The cuff should fit your arm snugly, yet smoothly.

Your arm should *not* be dangling at your side when your pressure is taken, but neither should it be held up in the air or randomly placed. Instead, the health care practitioner should gently support your arm, holding it out at the level of your heart. Any restrictive clothing or items such as purses should be removed.

The mercury column or gauge should be at the health care practitioner's eye level, or it can be misread.

After inflating the cuff to the point where the sounds are no longer heard through the stethoscope, the doctor or nurse should deflate the cuff *slowly*, no faster than 3 mm Hg per second. The point is to listen for subtle changes in sound, not be the first to finish.

When the first blood pressure reading has been completed, the doctor or nurse should wait a minute or two before taking a second one, if necessary.

By the way, the first time your health care practitioner examines you, he or she should take your blood pressure *three times*: once in the right arm, once in the left arm, and once in either thigh. Sometimes there will be discrepancies in the readings, suggesting vascular or other problems that should be looked into.

You can also have your blood pressure checked by automatic blood-pressure-checking machines at some gyms, pharmacies, or health fairs. These extra readings can be helpful between visits to your health care practitioner but should not take the place of your practitioner's regular monitoring. Remember:

These readings are not always accurate. The machines may misread your blood pressure. They may not be well maintained or hold your arm in the proper position. Gyms, pharmacies, and health fairs can also be noisy, which in itself may push your pressure up a little bit.

Step 2: Adopt the Specially Modified DASH Diet

A good diet can go a long way toward helping you maintain proper vascular tone and health. In fact, if you have stage 1 hypertension, you may be able to control your blood pressure simply by following the DASH diets (I and II).

The DASH diets can do more than lower your blood pressure. Because they're based on fruits, vegetables, and whole grains, the DASH diets can also help to reduce total cholesterol and LDL ("bad") cholesterol, thus lowering your risk of suffering a heart attack or stroke. And because the DASH does away with much of the processed, sugary foods we eat too much of, it may also help you control your weight, reduce insulin resistance, and hold diabetes at bay.

The DASH diet plus sodium restriction, known as the DASH-II diet, may lower your blood pressure even more than the original DASH-I diet, especially if you are sodium-sensitive.

See Chapter 5 for a detailed explanation of the modified DASH diet I use with my patients.

Step 3: Use the VasoGuard Therapy

For some people, the DASH or DASH-II diet alone will do the trick. Others, however, may have high blood pressure that requires more of a push before it will drop down to normal levels. You can get that extra assist from the supplements that make up the VasoGuard Therapy.

Take the supplements listed below twice a day. As your blood pressure falls, you and your physician can work together to start to decrease any antihypertensive medications you may be taking.

Mixed omega-3s (DHA and EPA)	2 gm
Celery seed powder	500 mg
Potassium (as citrate)	20 mcg
Vitamin B_6	100 mg
Natural mixed vitamin E	200 IU
Vitamin C (as calcium ascorbate)	500 mg
Garlic powder	250 mg
Taurine	1,500 mg
Natural lycopene tomato extract	1 mg
Biotin	800 mcg
CoEnzyme Q_{10} (Q-gel®)	50 mg
Lipoic acid	100 mg
Magnesium (as carbonate/sulfate)	185 mg
Calcium (as sulfate, rather than citrate or carbonate)	400 mg

You can purchase these supplements individually in most vitamin or health food stores, as well as many pharmacies and grocery stores. I am conducting ongoing clinical research on the effects of this formula and other dietary supplements on hypertension. For updates, go to the American Nutraceutical Association website at www.ana-jana.org.

In some cases, the VasoGuard Therapy may be all you need. Joan, a sixty-two-year-old former model, had high blood pressure despite exercising regularly and staying as slim as she was when she was modeling in her twenties and thirties. Her blood pressure was only moderately elevated, so we didn't have to rush right into medications. Instead, we took a good look at her eating habits and found that the various diets she had experimented with left her deficient in several vitamins and minerals. It's well known that a lack of common minerals such as calcium, magnesium, and potassium can cause or contribute to hypertension. Luckily, it's easy to solve this problem with supplements and a healthful diet. And that's exactly what happened.

Caution: The VasoGuard Therapy may be the most exciting part of the Hypertension Institute Program, *but this special combination of nutraceuticals is only one part of the program. It's tempting think you can get away with just popping a few pills, but that's not good enough. Even if the supplements bring your blood pressure down, you can do better by adopting the modified DASH diet and the other points in my program.*

Step 4: Exercise Regularly

Some people with hypertension shy away from exercise, fearing it will raise their blood pressure. It's true that exercise may increase your blood pressure, but only temporarily. Over time, a good exercise program will make your heart more efficient and improve your vascular tone, thus *lowering* your blood pressure.

We'll look at how exercise can help you in Chapter 7, as well as discuss which exercises are best and how you can safely begin your program.

Step 5: Maintain Your Ideal Weight

Obesity, all by itself, is a well-known risk factor for hypertension. Simply dropping those excess pounds can help bring your blood pressure down to a safer level. Losing weight can also help reduce your risk of developing diabetes, strokes, heart attacks, cancer, and other serious ailments. And the more weight you lose, the easier it will be to exercise.

Weight loss was all it took for forty-five-year-old Dawn to drop her blood pressure from 140/90 to 122/83. Alarmed when told that she had hypertension, this mother of three approached her weight loss program "like an athlete training for the Olympics." She dropped the twenty-five excess pounds she had been carrying around for years, and with the weight went the elevation in blood pressure. Now it's right around normal—and she didn't have to take any medications.

In Chapter 5 we'll look at ways to lose weight while following the DASH diet.

Step 6: De-stress Your Life

Numerous studies have linked stress, anxiety, fear, and other negative emotions to an elevation in blood pressure. Conversely, as stress decreases, so does blood pressure.

If you're like fifty-two-year-old James, you know when stress is pushing up your pressure. "I'm a contract negotiator for the movie studios," he explained. "Fighting is what I do for a living. Screaming, hollering, slamming the phone down—it's all in a day's work for me." Unfortunately, all that stress sent his blood pressure sky-high. James took stress-reduction and anger-management classes and took them seriously. He didn't want to "die and leave a widow and not-yet-grown-up kids behind." Over the course of a year or so, while we carefully monitored the situation, he learned to control himself while negotiating—and his pressure dropped down to the high normal range. "I found that I can negotiate without screaming, and live longer because of it. It's a win-win situation."

We'll look at ways to de-stress your life in Chapter 8.

Step 7: Reduce Your Alcohol Intake to a Reasonable Level

Excessive consumption of alcohol raises blood pressure and increases your risk of stroke. Chronic intake of more than 20 grams of alcohol a day (about the amount found in two drinks) increases the odds of developing hypertension, as well as the severity of the disease. Alcohol also interferes with your body's ability to absorb magnesium and zinc, which it needs to keep blood pressure within normal limits.

If you have hypertension, it's safest to set alcohol aside permanently. But if you do drink, your absolute maximum consumption should be less than 20 grams per day—that's about the amount of alcohol you'll find in 24 ounces of beer *or* 10 ounces of wine *or* 2 ounces of hard liquor. It's even better to limit yourself to less than 12 ounces of beer *or* 5 ounces of wine *or* 1 ounce of hard liquor.

We'll talk more about alcohol in Chapter 6.

Step 8: Cut Back on the Caffeine

The link between caffeine and hypertension is tenuous and controversial. Some studies show that caffeine raises blood pressure, while others say it doesn't. The confusion might be based on the fact that there are certain caffeine-sensitive people who show a blood pressure increase upon ingestion of this additive. And then there are those who show no change in blood pressure. What we do know is that caffeine is a stimulant that might push your pressure up, so it's best to limit yourself to moderate amounts.

I recommend an intake of less than 100 mg of caffeine per day, or about the amount in a 6-ounce cup of brewed coffee, 2½ cups of black tea, or two 12-ounce cans of a caffeinated soft drink. (But it's best to reduce or completely eliminate soft drink consumption.)

We'll talk more about caffeine in Chapter 6.

Step 9: Say Goodbye to Smoking and Tobacco

According to the American Heart Association, smoking accounts for over 430,000 deaths every year.[1] Giving up cigarettes and other forms of tobacco is tough because nicotine is extremely addicting. But it can be done. And it *must* be done, because all forms of tobacco contribute to endothelial dysfunction, hypertension, coronary heart disease, and other serious problems. Smoking is a major risk factor for heart disease, stroke, lung cancer, and other terrible ailments. It also reduces the protection against cardiovascular disease normally provided by antihypertensive therapy. In other words, you can work hard to lower your blood pressure, but if you smoke, you'll be negating much of the good that you've done. It's never too late to quit, and as soon as you do, your health will begin to improve. In fact, you'll see cardiovascular benefits within one year, no matter what your age.

Here are a few tips, adapted from the American Heart Association's recommendations, to help you stop smoking:

- Make a list of all the reasons you want to give up your cigarettes or other tobacco products.
- Read the list every day.
- Wrap the list around your cigarette pack, tape or clip it to

your box of cigarettes or your snuff container. If you want to smoke or chew tobacco, read that list before giving in to the urge.

- Think about every cigarette or cigar you smoke, every chaw of tobacco. Is it really important? Are you dying for it? If not, skip it.
- Cut back, little by little.
- Set up brief "no tobacco" periods for yourself. Try going without it for an hour, two hours, half a day, and so on.
- Make it a little tougher to smoke or chew tobacco. Don't carry matches with you, don't keep extra cartons of cigarettes, boxes of cigars, or containers of tobacco handy.
- When you feel like smoking or chewing, try exercising instead. Play a game, or find your loved one and have sex. Or why not transform your desire to please yourself through smoking into an opportunity to help others: Instead of sitting down to smoke on the weekend, go to a nearby senior center and volunteer your services.
- If possible, avoid the places where you usually smoke. Instead of the smoky bar, go to a nonsmoking restaurant.
- If you've given up tobacco, then slip and find yourself smoking or chewing again, don't kick yourself. Remember that you've got a tough habit to break, and it may take some time.

If you can give up tobacco by yourself, great. If not, don't feel embarrassed, for there's wisdom in asking for help. There are many good smoking cessation programs available, and your health care practitioner can help you get a nicotine transdermal patch, nicotine gum or Wellbutrin to help you ease off the real stuff. (The lower amounts of nicotine contained in smoking cessation aids usually will not raise blood pressure.)

You can get online information about nicotine patches, nicotine gum, or smoking cessation from organizations such as the American Heart Association (www.americanheart.org).

Step 10: Use Standard Medicines as Necessary

The VasoGuard Program can lower elevated blood pressure—and keep it down—for most people, most of the time. But there may be times when your pressure rises to dangerous levels and you'll need to take standard medicines for a while. Don't fight it! The right medication taken in the right amount can be a lifesaver, especially in times of emergency.

You'll find descriptions of the blood pressure medications, their uses, benefits, and side effects, in Chapter 9.

NEW AND OLD COMBINED

While my VasoGuard Program is new and revolutionary, the rest of the *Hypertension Institute Program* is grounded in the best of traditional medicine, incorporating the standard recommendations made by the American Heart Association, the Seventh Joint National Committee on Prevention, Detection, Evaluation, and Treatment of High Blood Pressure, the World Health Organization, and other prestigious health associations. But the various nutraceuticals recommended in this book are also grounded in the best of traditional medicine, put to the test in a variety of scientifically valid studies, justifying their use in my natural, safe, and gentle approach to controlling high blood pressure.

Now that we've learned about the program in general, it's time to delve into the particulars, beginning with the DASH diet.

Chapter 5

The DASH Diet

You may not feel much like a cave man (or cave woman), but your genetic makeup is practically identical to those who roamed the earth back then. Yet, if you're like most of us, your diet and lifestyle are a far cry from those of our ancient ancestors. We've "evolved" from hunter-gatherers who get plenty of exercise and consume a diet high in fiber, potassium, and omega-3 fatty acids, low in sodium and saturated fat, with moderate amounts of protein, unrefined carbohydrates, and calories, to couch potatoes who eat lots of unnatural, highly processed foods containing large amounts of saturated and trans fat, sodium, protein, and refined carbohydrates, and very little in the way of omega-3 fatty acids, vitamins, or minerals like potassium, calcium, and magnesium. We're paying the price with our health. Nutritionally related diseases like hypertension, diabetes, coronary heart disease, congestive heart failure, cancer, obesity, and hyperlipidemia (high blood fats) have hit epidemic levels in the United States. And unless we drastically change our ways, we can expect more of the same.

Luckily, we have the power to change things. The old saying by Hippocrates, "Food is your best medicine," has never been more relevant than it is today. This is particularly true with respect to hypertension, a disease that can be triggered or made much worse by a poor diet. The good news is that, in many cases, improving your diet can significantly reduce your elevated blood pressure, and even reverse its ill effects. In fact, you may be able to bring your blood pressure back down to normal levels *just by changing your diet.* And even if diet isn't the sole solution to your problem, it's certainly a vital part of any plan to combat hypertension.

THE FIRST DASH DIET

We've known for decades that vegetarians have lower blood pressure levels than nonvegetarians—an average of 10 to 15 mm Hg lower—and that they tend to develop hypertension less often. They also seem to avoid developing the steep rise in systolic blood pressure that we see so often in the rest of the population. And the stricter the vegetarian diet, the lower the blood pressure levels. Researchers began to wonder what it was about eating lots of vegetables and fruits that had positive effects on blood pressure. They decided to do studies on single nutrients to see if any one of them might be the magic bullet. But after several trials, the results seemed inconclusive. That is, the various nutrients were all helpful, but none seemed to stand head and shoulders above the others.

Perhaps, they thought, the whole is greater than the sum of the parts. Maybe single nutrients with only modest effects would produce much greater effects when combined with others. With this in mind, in 1997 the National Heart, Lung, and Blood Institute funded research on the effects on blood pressure of groups of nutrients as they're found together in foods. The name of this study was Dietary Approaches to Stop Hypertension, or DASH for short.

The DASH-I study was performed on 459 adults with untreated systolic blood pressures less than 159 mm Hg, and diastolic pressures between 80 and 95 mm Hg. This means that some of the subjects had normal blood pressure; in fact, only about 27 percent had hypertension. Males and females were represented about equally, and 60 percent of the subjects were African-American.

Three diets were used:

- a control diet similar to the standard American diet
- a diet similar to the standard American diet, plus more fruits and vegetables
- the DASH-I diet, which is high in fruits, vegetables, and low-fat dairy products, but low in cholesterol, saturated fat, and total fat

Each of these three diets contained about 3,000 mg of sodium, an average amount for many Americans. The diets were randomly assigned to the subjects, who were then followed for a period of eight weeks. During the study period, the subjects didn't try to lower their sodium intake, lose weight, or exercise any more than normal.

At the end of the trial, both the fruits and vegetables group and the DASH-I diet group showed marked reductions in blood pressure. This demonstrated that simply eating more fruits and vegetables is helpful.

But those on the DASH-I diet enjoyed the greatest drop in their systolic and diastolic pressure. And the drop in blood pressure took place earlier than it did in the other group—

starting as soon as the diet was begun, reaching maximum levels at about two weeks. The most dramatic results were seen in the hypertensive subjects following the DASH-I diet, who had blood pressure reductions of nearly 11 mm Hg systolic and 5.5 mm Hg diastolic.[1] The researchers were thrilled because these results were just as good as those seen with medications for mild hypertension.

THE DASH-II DIET

Buoyed by this success, the researchers soon set to work on a second study. Knowing that lowering sodium intake can help decrease blood pressure, they decided to test a combination of the DASH diet plus sodium restriction against the standard American diet. This study was called the DASH-II Sodium (or DASH-II for short); the first one was renamed DASH-I to distinguish between the two. The DASH-II study involved 412 subjects with systolic blood pressures ranging between 129 and 159 mm Hg, and diastolic pressures of 80 to 95 mm Hg. About 57 percent were African-American, 57 percent were women, and 41 percent were hypertensive. Half of the subjects were randomly assigned the DASH-II diet, the other half the standard American diet. Each subject also consumed a specific level of sodium for one month at a time: 4,300 mg per day during the first month; 2,400 mg/day during the second month; and 1,500 mg per day during the third month.

The results showed that simply cutting back on sodium intake reduced the blood pressure, whether subjects were on the DASH-II diet or the standard American diet. But those on the DASH-II diet showed greater reductions in blood pressure at each level. Again, the greatest reductions in blood pressure were seen in hypertensives, especially those who were on the

DASH-II diet with sodium levels restricted to 1,500 mg. But significant decreases were also seen in those *with normal blood pressure* who followed this combination plan.

MORE SUPPORT FOR THE DASH

The validity of the DASH-I and DASH-II diets was recently boosted by the results of the Vanguard Study.[2] For this randomized study, volunteers were divided into two groups:

- The at-risk group consisted of seventy-one people with untreated hypertension or hypertension plus hyperlipidemia (elevated triglycerides and cholesterol). They were given a special diet similar to the DASH-I.
- The healthy group consisted of eighty-seven people who had normal blood pressures, cholesterol, and blood fats. They consumed diets they created themselves after receiving nutritional counseling.

After ten weeks on the diets, both systolic and diastolic blood pressure had fallen an average of 2 mm Hg in those eating the do-it-yourself diets, but an even more impressive 8 mm Hg systolic and 5 mm Hg diastolic in those on the DASH-I-like diet.

The Vanguard Study is one of many recent trials[3] that have studied the use of nutrients that occur naturally in whole foods to lower elevated blood pressure, as opposed to using isolated components of the diet (for example, using a whole apple instead of just the vitamin C from that same apple).

The message from these studies is clear: *You can lower your blood pressure significantly by following the DASH-I diet and restricting your sodium intake to 1,500 mg per day, or less. And you can expect to see results that are equal to those achieved through monodrug therapy for mild hypertension.* These results are immediate, sustainable, and inexpensive. This diet can improve your nutrient status *and* your quality of life. If you do nothing else that I recommend in this book, do this! It may be enough all by itself.

WARNING!

If you're currently taking medication to control your high blood pressure, *do not use the diet in lieu of your medicine*. Talk to your health care practitioner before making any changes in your medication intake.

MODIFYING THE DASH

The DASH-I and DASH-II diets have proven their value in studies and in the lives of many people suffering from hypertension. Good as the two DASH diets are, however, they can be made even better with subtle tweaking to reduce the amount of simple carbohydrates and increase the "good" fat and protein. At my Hypertension Institute, I give my patients a specially modified version of the DASH that I believe is the best diet possible for people with hypertension. The main change is to increase the amount of protein, vegetables, and "good" fats consumed every day, while decreasing the grains, fruits, and dairy products. Otherwise, it's the same great, pressure-reducing program that has helped so many.

Here's what the modified DASH diet is made of:

Food Group	Number of Servings	Serving Size	Suggestions
Cereal, grains, pasta	3–4 per day	1 oz dry flax or whole grain cereal, ½ cup cooked cereal, 1 slice bread, ½ cup cooked whole wheat pasta	Eat whole grain breads, cereals, and pastas with no added sugar or salt.
Vegetables	8–10 per day	1 medium, 1 cup raw (chopped), ½ cup cooked 6 oz unprocessed fresh vegetable juice	Eat your vegetables raw, or cook them lightly without adding salt or fats. You can substitute vegetable juice for *one serving* per day, but make sure it contains no salt.
Fruits	2–3 per day	1 medium, 1 cup raw (chopped), ½ cup cooked	Eat your fruits raw whenever possible. If chopped, cut just before serving to preserve all the vitamins.
Meat, Poultry, Fish	2–4 per day	3–5 oz cooked	Lean cuts only; trim fat; skin poultry. Coldwater fish preferred.
Dried beans, seeds, nuts	1–2 per day	½ cup cooked beans, 2 tbsp seeds, ⅓ cup nuts, 3 oz tofu	Choose unsalted nuts or seeds. Avoid canned beans because of high-sodium/sugar content.
Dairy	1–2 per day	1 cup nonfat or low-fat milk, buttermilk, or yogurt; 1½ oz nonfat or low-fat cheese (low-sodium kind)	Dairy products are great sources of calcium, but also provide moderate amounts of sodium. Get the low-fat or nonfat and low-sodium varieties whenever possible.

The DASH Diet

Food Group	Number of Servings	Serving Size	Suggestions
Fats, oils	4–5 per day	1 tsp canola mayonnaise, 1 tsp olive oil, 1 tsp spread made from omega-3 fatty acids	Reduce saturated fat. Replace with monounsaturated oils, such as canola or olive oil.
Sweets	None		Avoid candy, pastries, sugar, honey, syrup, and jelly.

THAT'S A LOT OF FRUITS AND VEGETABLES!

As you can see, the DASH-I menu probably has more servings of fruits, vegetables, and grains than you're currently eating, and less meat, fish, and poultry. Although it's really quite a pleasant way to eat, it might take some getting used to if you're hooked on the standard American burgers-fries-cola diet. Most people don't have too much trouble adding grains to their diets—just eat another slice of whole wheat bread or a double portion of whole grain cereal. But adding several servings of vegetables and fruits can be another matter. To make sure you're getting enough, try the following:

• Add a glass of grapefruit juice to your breakfast. That's an easy way to increase your fruit intake.

• Top off your breakfast with some whole fruit. Try a sliced apple or ½ cup of berries on your cereal.

• Slip a couple of slices of tomato into your sandwich.

• Chop up some raw vegetables, put them in a plastic bag, and take them to work with you. They make great snacks.

• Saute some sliced mushrooms in a tablespoon of chicken broth for an elegant side dish.

- For a delicious, satisfying, low-fat dessert, freeze 1 cup washed, stemmed strawberries for 30 minutes, then place them in a blender with ¼ cup low-fat yogurt and blend.
- Begin your lunch or dinner with a big, raw vegetable salad. Then move on to the meat, fish, or poultry dish.
- Make a smoothie from 1 cup of chopped blueberries blended with 1 cup nonfat yogurt.
- Homemade vegetable soup, vegetarian chili, meatless curry, and veggie stir-fry are all delicious easy ways to get more vegetables into your diet.

HOLD THE SALT!

The DASH-II diet is just like the DASH-I, plus sodium restrictive. You've undoubtedly heard that salt (sodium chloride) can be dangerous for hypertensives. Although this is often the case, it's not true for everyone. We can't give an exact figure, but we estimate that up to 60 percent of those with elevated blood pressure are salt-sensitive. That is, their blood pressure rises when they consume more salt, and falls when they take in less. We also know that African-Americans, the elderly, and the obese are more likely to be salt-sensitive, and that there may be a genetic component to this susceptibility.

Whether you're salt-sensitive or not, you can expect your blood pressure to fall when you go on the DASH-II diet, as outlined above. But cutting back on your sodium intake may help you push your blood pressure down even more. This is probably because sodium increases your blood volume, which raises your pressure—especially if you're salt-sensitive.

When sodium restriction was added to the DASH-I diet (the DASH-II trials), the average blood pressure reduction in hypertensives was 11.5 mm Hg systolic and 6.8 mm Hg diastolic. And the more that sodium was restricted, the lower the pressure went. Clearly, the very best way to lower your pressure is to follow the DASH-II diet, which includes at least a moderate restriction of sodium.

The typical sodium intake in the U.S. is between 6 and 10 grams per day (the equivalent of about 3 to 5 teaspoons of salt). And in some areas of the country, people consume 15,000 to 20,000 mg per day, or up to nearly 10 teaspoons of the stuff. Our actual physiological need for sodium is more like 500 mg per day—about as much as is found in ¼ teaspoon. (The need is probably slightly higher if you exercise heavily and lose sodium through perspiration.)

I hesitate to tell people to cut back on sodium too severely, especially at first, since an extremely low-sodium diet can be hard to follow for very long, and severe sodium restriction (less than 500 mg per day) can actually lead to dehydration. So I usually recommend an intake of between 1,500 mg and 2,000 mg. In this range, most people will see their blood pressures fall, yet their food can still taste good.

Sodium Isn't Just Salt

In order to cut back on your sodium intake effectively, you'll have to become a bit of a detective. There's often plenty of sodium lurking in processed, packaged, and canned foods, although you might not recognize it at first glance. The biggest offenders are:

- *Salt*—Seventy-five percent of our sodium intake comes from processed foods, and the rest from salt added to our food in cooking and at the table. So maybe it's time to pack away your salt shaker. If you're just not ready for that, try substituting potassium chloride for salt. You can find No-Salt and other potassium chloride brands in grocery stores or health food stores. By the way, when you use potassium chloride instead of salt, you're helping to normalize your blood pressure in two ways at once: First, you're cutting back on your sodium, and second, you're consuming more potassium. (You need to consume at least 2,400 mg potassium per day to have a beneficial effect.)

- *Brine*—This is a saltwater solution used for pickling and preserving. Watch out for a high-sodium content in pickled foods, canned vegetables, canned meats or fish packed in saltwater, and packaged seafood.
- *MSG (monosodium glutamate)*—MSG is an unnecessary additive found in everything from ketchup to Chinese food. When you eat out, ask the waiter if the restaurant uses MSG and request that they leave it out of your food. At home, there's no need to use it: Just add more spices if you want more taste.
- *Baking soda (sodium bicarbonate)*—If you've ever brushed your teeth with this, you know it's salty! Avoid commercial baked goods or packaged mixes, for they often contain baking soda. Grain products made with small amounts of baking soda and baking powder are all right, in moderation.
- *Baking powder (sodium aluminum sulfate)*—If you do your own baking, you can substitute potassium bicarbonate for baking powder.

Either eliminate or severely limit any foods with these ingredients. You should also beware of any foods that contain the following:

- Disodium phosphate
- Sodium alginate
- Sodium benzoate
- Sodium hydroxide
- Sodium propionate
- Sodium saccharin
- Sodium sulfite

High-Sodium Foods

Here's a partial list of high-sodium foods to avoid:

Baking powder*
Baking soda
Barbecue sauce
Bouillon cubes*
Buttermilk*
Celery, dehydrated
Celery salt
Cereal, instant
Cheese (most)*
Cottage cheese*
Crackers*
Fish, canned, smoked, breaded*
Frozen dinners
Garlic salt
Horseradish, prepared
Ketchup*
Lemon-pepper marinade
Meat extracts
Meats, canned, smoked, cured
Meats, Kosher
Meat tenderizer*
Monosodium glutamate (MSG)
Mustard, prepared*
Nuts, salted*
Olives*
Onion salt
Parsley flakes
Party spreads and dips
Peanut butter*
Pickles*
Popcorn, salted*
Potato chips, corn chips*
Pretzels*
Relish
Rennet tablets
Salad dressing, bottled or dry mix
Salt
Sauerkraut
Sausage
Soups, canned or packaged
Soy sauce*
Steak sauce
Teriyaki sauce*
Vegetable juice, canned*
Worcestershire sauce*

*Low-sodium versions can be purchased.

High-Sodium Medications

You might not realize it, but certain over-the-counter medications contain high levels of sodium, so always check the labels for sodium content. Some common medications that contain sodium include:

- Alka-Seltzer
- Bromo-Seltzer
- Gelusil liquid
- Maalox suspension
- Metamucil instant mix
- Mylanta-II liquid
- Rolaids

Low-sodium equivalents of these medications are available in most cases. Ask your doctor or pharmacist for recommendations.

What *Can* You Eat When You're Watching Your Sodium Intake?

You may think that if you avoid all of the foods on the high-sodium list, there will be nothing left worth eating! But there are plenty of delicious foods that contain low to moderate amounts of sodium and are allowed on a sodium-restricted diet:

Cereal, Grains, Pasta
  Unsalted grains or noodles, shredded wheat, matzoh, corn tortillas, puffed rice, unsalted popcorn, yeast breads (up to 3 servings a day).

Vegetables
Fresh, frozen, or canned without added salt. Vegetable juice without added salt.

Fruits
Fresh, frozen, or canned without added salt or sugars.

Meat, Poultry, Fish
Fresh, unsalted, or canned meat, poultry, or fish. Unsalted vegetarian meat analog products.

Dried Beans, Seeds, Nuts
Unsalted nuts or seeds, unsalted dried beans, tofu.

Dairy
Milk, unsalted buttermilk, low-sodium cheese (e.g., Swiss, ricotta, Gruyère), regular and frozen yogurt.

Soup
Homemade soup (limit added salt), low-sodium canned soup.

Fats and Oils
Preferably unsalted or low-sodium omega-3 spread or canola mayonnaise. Olive oil and vinegar or lemon for salad dressing.

Seasonings
Herbs, spices, garlic, lemon juice, onion, Tabasco sauce, pepper, vinegar, fresh-ground horseradish, oils, extracts of vanilla, peppermint, lemon. Watch out for seasonings made of meat and vegetable extracts. If no packaged, processed, or

canned foods are used, you may use ¼ teaspoon of table salt per day.

Tips for Slashing Your Sodium Intake

- Get rid of your salt shaker and don't add salt to foods when you're cooking.
- If you're having trouble adjusting to the no-added-salt philosophy, begin by cutting in half the amount of salt you'd normally use. Then cut it in half again a week later. Continue until you've stopped adding salt.
- Remember that most of the salt and sodium we consume comes from processed foods. Read your food labels and try to eliminate as many processed foods as possible.
- Try lemon juice and fresh ground pepper to bring out the flavor of poultry or fish.
- Rinse the contents of canned foods (tuna, for instance) with water to remove some of the sodium.
- Use reduced-sodium or no-salt-added versions of foods and condiments (mustard, ketchup, pickles, sauces).
- Treat low-sodium soy sauce the same way you'd treat added salt: Use very sparingly.
- Watch out for multi-ingredient dishes like pizza or frozen dinners, as they're very high in sodium.
- Try spices instead of salt. You'll find you can taste the food better.
- These terms should throw up a red flag: cured, pickled, soy sauce, broth, meat extract, bouillon.

Spicing It Up!

When you're trying to cut back on salt, herbs and spices can be your best friends. Take a look at how you can use some of the herbs and spices that are probably sitting in your cupboard right now:

- *Basil*—Add ½ tsp to 2 tbsp olive oil and use for basting fish or chicken during baking; ½ tsp to 2 cups green vegetables while steaming; ¾ tsp to 1 lb ground beef or chicken when making meatloaf or patties for grilling.
- *Chili powder*—Add 1 tbsp to vegetarian chili during simmering; sprinkle ½ tsp over 4 cups popcorn; sprinkle 1 tsp chili powder, 1 tbsp lime juice, and ⅓ cup chopped raw onion over baked fish fillets.
- *Curry powder*—Add 1½ tsp to 2 cups cooked brown rice in the final stages of cooking; 2 tsp to 2 cups vegetables simmered in low-sodium tomato sauce; 1½ tsp to stir-fry chicken and vegetables.
- *Dill weed*—Mix 1 tsp with 1 tbsp low-fat, low-sodium margarine. Spread over hot bread or freshly cooked noodles. Add ½ tsp to 2 cups freshly steamed green beans.
- *Mint*—Chop fresh leaves and add to peas while cooking. Use as a garnish for fresh fruit salad.
- *Nutmeg*—Add ½ tsp to 2 cups cooked carrots; sprinkle over fresh fruit cup; mix ⅛ tsp into 1 lb ground chicken before cooking.
- *Oregano*—Mix 1 tsp with 1 tbsp melted low-fat, low-sodium margarine and use as a baste for fish or chicken. Sprinkle over fresh vegetable salad. Add 1 to 2 tsp to cooked noodles.
- *Rosemary*—Add 1 to 2 tsp to ground chicken or beef be-

fore making into patties. Sprinkle ½ tsp over baked potato. Add ½ tsp to flour before dredging 3 lb chicken.

- *Tarragon*—Add ¼ tsp to sautéed mushrooms; add 1 tsp to 1 lb ground chicken; sprinkle over deviled eggs made with low-fat mayonnaise.

SHED THOSE EXCESS POUNDS

Scientists have long known that obesity and high blood pressure go hand in hand. And for many people, losing weight is absolutely the most effective technique for lowering blood pressure. Too much fat, especially if it settles around your waist, not only drives up your blood pressure, but also puts you at a much higher risk for heart disease, stroke, Type II diabetes, osteoarthritis of the weight-bearing joints, and certain cancers.

How can you tell definitively if you're overweight? A general rule of thumb is if your waist measurement is greater than 35 inches, for women, or 40 inches, for men, or if your BMI (body mass index) is greater than 25, then you're most likely overweight.

CALCULATING YOUR BMI

Your body mass index (BMI) is calculated by dividing your body weight (in kilograms) by your height (in meters) squared. An easier way to figure this is:
- Multiply your weight in pounds by 0.45 (e.g., if you weigh 120, multiply by 0.45 and you get 54).

- Multiply your height in inches by 0.025 (if you're 5'4", you're 64 inches tall: 64 x 0.025 = 1.6).
- Multiply your answer from step 2 by itself (1.6 x 1.6 = 2.56).
- Divide your answer from step 1 by your answer from step 3 (54 ÷ 2.56 = 21.09375, which rounds off to 21).
- Your BMI is 21.

If your BMI is greater than 25, you need to do something about your weight—now!

Note: The BMI is not an accurate gauge of obesity or overfatness for certain people. A professional football player or a wrestler, for example, may weigh a lot and have a high BMI. But much of that weight is due to muscle, not fat, so in spite of the high BMI, this person is not overweight or overfat. On the other hand, some very skinny models may have lower BMIs but still may be overly fatty. Why? Because the small amount of "meat" on their bones is primarily fat, not muscle. So relative to their weight, they have too much fat and not enough muscle. Pro football players, ballerinas, and others may need more than the BMI to determine whether or not they're overweight or overfat. For most of us, however, the BMI is right on target.

How Those Extra Pounds Drive Up Your Blood Pressure

Why does excess weight cause hypertension? First and foremost, fat is living tissue that needs a blood supply to deliver nutrients and haul away the wastes. It's been estimated that it takes a mile of capillaries to service one pound of fat—an extra mile of blood vessels through which your heart has to pump blood. When you multiply that by 20, 30, 50, or 100 pounds of extra fat, you've added a huge amount to your heart's workload.

Excess weight also contributes to *insulin resistance*. Insulin is a hormone that helps blood glucose enter numerous body cells, where it's used as fuel. Insulin acts like a key that fits into an imaginary lock called an *insulin receptor site* in the cell membranes. Once insulin unlocks this door to the cell, the glucose can enter. But without enough insulin, many cells remain locked up and can't receive their food. Then, even though the vital glucose in the bloodstream may build up to sky-high levels, it will simply float on by, unable to enter and nourish the hungry cells. This happens when the body doesn't manufacture enough insulin, as in Type I diabetes.

But this starvation in the midst of plenty can also happen when the body makes plenty of insulin but the cells don't respond well to that insulin. If your cells are ignoring insulin's command to open up, you have the condition called insulin resistance. There's plenty of glucose and ample insulin, but for some reason the insulin can't unlock the cells, so the glucose just drifts on down the bloodstream. Why can't the glucose enter? Two reasons have to do with excess weight. Fat cells can block the insulin receptor sites (the locks) on cell membranes, making it impossible for the insulin to do its job. And fat cells themselves can be insulin-resistant. So the more fat cells you have, the more you'll be plagued by insulin resistance.

Naturally, the body is unhappy that the glucose is not being escorted into the cells by the insulin. So the pancreas pumps out even more insulin, trying to make the cells open up and accept the glucose. That may do the trick; the extra insulin may force the glucose into the cells. This solves one problem, but creates another, for too much insulin in your system can be dangerous. Insulin increases sodium retention in the body, which increases blood volume and ratchets up your pressure. It also speeds atherosclerosis, making your blood vessels stiffer, narrower, and more resistant.

A Drop in Weight = A Drop in Blood Pressure

The good news is that, in many cases, all you need to do is lose weight to see immediate improvement in both insulin resistance and elevated blood pressure. In fact, weight loss is one of the most effective ways to reduce blood pressure significantly[4] in overweight hypertensives,[5] overweight people with high-normal blood pressure,[6] nonobese patients with hypertension, and nonobese patients with high normal pressure.[7]

And you don't have to get your weight all the way down to the ideal level in order to enjoy a lower pressure.[8] This was demonstrated in two key studies, the Trial of Hypertension Prevention I and II. In these studies, a weight loss of just under 10 pounds (4.4 kg) resulted in an average blood pressure reduction of 7 mm Hg systolic and 5 mm Hg diastolic. That may not sound like a lot, but remember that each reduction of 1 mm Hg in diastolic blood pressure reduces your risk of coronary heart disease by 3 percent and your risk of stroke by 7 percent. The effects of systolic blood pressure reduction are even more impressive.

Slimming down is essential, but beware. There are many unbalanced diets out there that may help you shed the pounds but will leave you short of calcium, potassium, and other substances you need to remain healthy and keep your blood pressure under control. Avoid crash and crazy diets like the plagues they are.

Dieting with DASH

If you eat the recommended number of servings on the DASH diet (either DASH-I or DASH-II), you'll take in approximately 2,000 calories per day. If you're significantly overweight or fairly active, there's a fair chance you consume more than 2,000 calories per day, so simply adopting the DASH will be like going on a weight loss diet.

If, on the other hand, you're very sedentary, weigh less than 150 pounds, or are only slightly overweight, you may already be eating 2,000 or fewer calories per day. In that case, you may need to drop down to a 1,600-calorie-per-day diet. You can still lose weight with either DASH diet by eating a lower number of the recommended servings.

Here's how you can adapt the modified DASH diet to about 1,600 calories per day:

1,600 Calorie DASH Diet

Cereal, grains, pasta	3 servings per day
Vegetables	8 servings per day
Fruits	2 servings per day
Meat, poultry, fish	2 servings per day
Dried beans, seeds, nuts	1 serving per day
Dairy	2 servings per day
Fats, oils	4 servings per day
Sweets	0 per day

If you follow these basic guidelines, you can consume the diet proven to lower elevated blood pressure while simultaneously losing weight. And since the mere act of losing weight helps reduce blood pressure, you'll be attacking the problem from two angles at once.

PUTTING IT ALL TOGETHER

I find that the best way to think about the DASH diet is to visualize our good old ancestor, Paleolithic man, and try to emulate his ways. There he is, striding through the woods, eating berries and root vegetables as he finds them. Maybe he gets lucky and spears a wild animal on the run, so he can have a small amount of lean meat along with his vegetables and fruits for dinner. He's never had any added salt, and he doesn't need it. As for preservatives or other food processing—forget it! He eats what nature provides and, for the most part, eats it in its natural state. Whatever seasoning he adds comes from the herbs that grow nearby. That's what we're doing with the modified DASH: returning to a more natural way of eating so that we can get away from diet-induced hypertension and our bodies can return to normal, healthy functioning.

What does all this mean in terms of what you should eat every day? For many people, it means doubling their consumption of fruits and vegetables, cutting back on fat, and using low-fat or nonfat dairy products. (There's an added benefit to the DASH diet. Since you're not eating a lot of manufactured, processed foods, you'll probably see your food bill drop.) When translated to a sample day's menu, you might be eating something like this:

Breakfast
½ grapefruit
1 cup cooked oatmeal
1 cup green tea
1 cup blueberries
1 slice pumpernickel toast
1 tsp omega-3 spread

Lunch
　Turkey sandwich made with:
　　4–6 oz turkey, white meat, roasted without skin
　　2 tsp canola mayonnaise
　　2 slices whole wheat bread
　　a sprinkle of tarragon
　Raw vegetables, including:
　　1 cup broccoli
　　2 stalks celery
　　1 whole tomato
　　1½ cups raw mushrooms
　Vegetable dip made of:
　　Olive oil, vinegar, and chopped garlic
　1 orange
　1 cup low-fat frozen yogurt

Snack
　½ cup berries

Dinner
　4–6 oz grilled salmon
　1 cup baby lima beans
　Salad made with:
　　1 cup raw spinach
　　¼ cup chopped red onion
　　½ tomato, chopped
　　⅓ cup sliced cucumbers
　　2 tbsp olive-oil–based dressing
　1 piece pumpernickel bread
　1 cup green tea

Snack
　1 cup fresh cherries

IT ALL BEGINS WITH ONE STEP

If following the modified DASH diet sounds impossible, or at least a huge change, don't worry. You don't have to become a perfect lean, mean, eating machine overnight. Think of the DASH diet as the goalposts at the end of the football field. You just want to keep moving in that direction, no matter how long it takes to get there, no matter how many times you're tackled by salty, fatty, or processed foods.

Begin by increasing your servings of fruits, vegetables, and grains, and lowering your fat intake. Gradually cut back on your sodium, but not to the point where your food is tasteless. You'll probably find that your food is actually tastier once you ease up on the salt, and that fresh fruits and vegetables have subtle but delicious flavors that you weren't aware of in the past. Do the best you can, but if you should slip up and eat a non-DASH meal once in a while, relax! Just pick up where you left off and make sure your next meal puts you back on track.

The diet may be a DASH, but the technique is slow and steady. Eating right for life is a marathon, not a sprint. To help you get started on your new eating plan, here are a few examples of some delicious, heart-healthy, blood-pressure-lowering recipes.

RECIPES

Feel free to experiment and make up your own recipes. Just remember to increase your intake of fresh fruits and vegetables, whole grains, and foods rich in omega-3 fatty acids, while lowering your intake of sodium and saturated fat.

Breakfast Ideas

Scrambled Eggs with Spinach and Fresh Salsa

This breakfast is easy and nourishing, and you can increase the nutrient value of this dish by using omega-3-rich eggs, now available in your local grocery store.

Make the salsa first:

Salsa

1 bunch cilantro
¼ cup diced red onion
1 small seeded jalapeño pepper, minced
1 cup chopped fresh tomatoes
¼ cup chopped red pepper
2 tbsp freshly squeezed lime juice

Toss ingredients together until well blended. Cover and refrigerate until ready to use.

Scrambled Eggs

1 tsp olive oil
¼ cup sliced mushrooms
¼ cup sliced green onions
¼ cup chopped red pepper
¼ cup chopped green pepper
2 omega-3-rich eggs
1 tsp water
1 cup fresh spinach

Put olive oil in a medium-size nonstick frying pan and place over medium heat. Sauté the mushrooms, onions, and peppers for about 2 minutes; remove pan from heat. In a small bowl, beat together eggs and water. Return frying pan with vegetables to low heat and add egg mixture. Add fresh spinach leaves; mix thoroughly and cook for 2–3 minutes. Serve with the salsa. Makes 1 serving.

Health Nut Toast

Instead of eating ordinary buttered toast for breakfast, treat yourself to this easy-to-fix power-packed energy booster. Wheat germ, the embryo of the wheat berry, is loaded with thiamin, vitamin E, magnesium, and selenium. Almond butter is rich in potassium, magnesium, and monounsaturated fats. For a complete and highly nutritious meal, eat this toast with yogurt.

2 slices whole grain bread
2 tbsp almond butter
2 tbsp toasted wheat germ
½ cup fresh berries

Toast bread until lightly browned. While bread is still warm, spread 1 tbsp almond butter on each piece. Sprinkle with wheat germ and the ½ cup of berries. Makes 2 servings.

Entrées

Chicken Waldorf Salad Sandwich

This healthy twist on the crunchy salad made popular by the Waldorf-Astoria hotel is a surefire hit on picnics and in lunch boxes. It packs well and doesn't get soggy.

1 cup cooked, diced chicken breast
½ cup thinly sliced celery
½ cup sliced green or red grapes
½ cup chopped walnuts
½ cup diced peeled red apples
2 tsp canola oil
⅛ tsp black pepper
½ tsp celery seed
1 whole wheat pita bread, cut in half

Combine all ingredients and stuff into the pita halves. Another way to serve this salad is to spoon it into the hollowed-out halves of a cantaloupe or papaya, and eat the pita bread on the side. Either way, it's delicious. Makes 2 servings.

Smoked Turkey Wrap with Avocado

This tasty, vitamin-packed wrap goes well with a cup of soup or a fruit salad. Keep in mind that sprouts from nutrient-dense seeds like lentils, mung beans, or soybeans offer a broad range of nutraceuticals.

1 spinach or tomato basil tortilla
1 tbsp hummus
4 oz sliced low-sodium smoked turkey

½ small ripe avocado, peeled and sliced
½ cup sprouts (from mung beans, soybeans, lentils)
½ diced roma tomato
½ cup baby green lettuce

Lay tortilla on flat surface and spread hummus evenly in the middle. Top with turkey, avocado slices, sprouts, tomato, and lettuce. Starting on one end, begin to roll, folding the sides in as you go. The tighter you roll, the less likely that your wrap will fall apart. Makes 1 serving.

Mediterranean Veal Stew

A lower rate of heart disease is seen in Spain, Italy, southern France, and parts of the Middle East, where people typically consume plenty of red wine plus a diet high in monounsaturated fats, vegetables, fruits, fish, nuts, and seeds. Olives, wine, and pine nuts contribute a rich Mediterranean flair to this simple 30-minute stew.

2 tbsp extra virgin olive oil
1 lb lean veal stewing meat, trimmed of all visible fat and cut into 1½ inch cubes
4 cloves garlic, crushed
2 cups chopped yellow onion
1 cup red wine
2 cups chopped tomatoes
1 lb bag broccoli florets
1 cup fresh basil, minced
1 small can black olives, sliced
4 tbsp pine nuts
freshly ground black pepper

Heat olive oil in a skillet over medium heat. Brown the veal and remove from skillet. Add garlic and onion to skillet; sauté for 3 minutes, then add wine and cook for 1 minute. Reduce heat to medium-low, add tomatoes, broccoli, and veal. Cover and simmer for 20 minutes. Stir in fresh basil, olives, and pine nuts. Cook an additional 5 minutes. Season with pepper. Makes 4 servings. Serve with a spring mixed salad with raspberry vinaigrette dressing.

Tropical Roasted Salmon

Rich in heart-healthy omega-3s, salmon also provides loads of other nutrients, including protein, potassium, selenium, and an impressive amount of vitamin B_{12}. Fresh ginger, nutmeg, chili powder, and cumin turn this tasty fish into an extraordinary entrée.

4 (6 oz) salmon fillets
1 tsp freshly grated ginger
2 tbsp fresh lemon juice
1–2 tbsp extra virgin olive oil
4 tsp chili powder
2 tsp grated lemon rind
¾ tsp ground cumin
¼ tsp ground cinnamon
dash nutmeg
lemon wedges (optional)

Place salmon into a plastic baking bag; combine the fresh ginger, and lemon juice and pour over fish inside the bag. Seal bag and put in refrigerator to marinate for 1 hour, turning occasionally.

Preheat oven to 400 degrees. Remove fish from bag; discard marinade. Brush fillets lightly with olive oil. In a small bowl, combine chili powder, lemon rind, cumin, cinnamon, and nutmeg. Rub over fillets on both sides.

Place fish in a baking dish lightly coated with cooking spray. Bake 10–15 minutes, or until fish is cooked through and flakes easily when tested with a fork. Serve with lemon wedges, if desired. Makes 4 servings.

Smoothies

Smoothies make great breakfasts, afternoon pick-me-ups, or desserts. These smoothies are also loaded with beta-carotene, protein, flavonoids, pectin, vitamin C, and omega-3s. Using this recipe as inspiration, create your own smoothies.

Fruit Medley Smoothie

1 cup strawberries
1 ripe peach
8 oz soy milk
1 tsp flaxseed oil
1 cup crushed ice

Remove stems from strawberries and skin from peach. Place in blender. Pour in soy milk and blend until smooth. Add flaxseed oil and crushed ice. Blend again until mixture becomes thick and creamy. Makes 2 servings.

YOU *CAN* STICK TO IT

The few recipes I've given you are just a beginning. You can be creative as you like, or you can keep it simple. Some of my patients throw themselves into preparing elaborate, gourmet meals, while others are happy with bowls of whole grains, vegetable and fruit salads, and grilled fish or chicken. There is no right or wrong.

The only consideration is what works for you. Which approach, which recipes, will help you stay on the modified DASH diet forever. Remember, this isn't a quickie diet you stay on until your blood pressure drops down to safe levels, then you toss out the window. You're making a lifelong commitment to your good health. A commitment you should keep. A commitment you *can* keep.

Chapter 6

Design Your Own Diet

If you do nothing other than increase your fruit, vegetable, and grain servings, while lowering your sodium and fat intake, you'll be doing your body a huge favor. In other words, all you have to do is adopt the modified DASH diet and there's an excellent chance that you'll lower your blood pressure and reduce your risk of heart disease, stroke, Type II diabetes, and certain cancers (particularly those of the breast, prostate, and colon).

You may prefer, however, to create your own diet. If so, you can use the following list of helpful foods and supplements as a framework for designing your own antihypertensive eating plan.

GUIDELINES FOR CREATING YOUR OWN ANTI-HYPERTENSIVE DIET

The recommendations in the following list have been shown to be helpful for lowering elevated blood pressure. If you can incorporate all of them into your daily, do-it-yourself diet, great. If you can't, don't worry. Focus on items 1 through 9, the big guns for fighting hypertension.

1. *Sodium*—1,500–2,000 mg.
2. *Potassium*—2,400–4,000 mg.
3. *Potassium/sodium (P/S) ratio*—2:1 to 5:1 or greater if possible. Definitely make it more than 1:1.
4. *Magnesium*—500–1,000 mg.
5. *Calcium*—1,000–1,500 mg.
6. *Zinc*—25 mg.
7. *Protein*—1.0–1.2 grams per kilogram of body weight.
8. *Fats*—25–35 percent of your total calories should come from fats of all kinds: 10 percent in the form of omega-3 fatty PUFA; 10 percent omega-6 fatty PUFA; 50 percent omega-9 fatty acids MUFA; and less than 30 percent in the form of saturated fatty acids from lean and/or wild animal meat. The P/S ratio, or ratio of polyunsaturated to saturated fats, should be greater than 2:1. No trans fatty acids.
9. *Carbohydrates*—35 percent or less of your total calories should come from carbohydrates, preferably the complex carbohydrates found in whole grains, vegetables, beans, and legumes.
10. *Garlic*—4 cloves or 4 grams of garlic per day.
11. *Mushrooms*—Add shiitake and maitake mushrooms to your salads, stir frys, and so on.
12. *Guava fruit*—1–2 medium guavas.
13. *Wakame seaweed*—3–3 ½ grams (2 tablespoons) of dried wakame seaweed per day.
14. *Celery*—Your choice of: 4 stalks per day, 8 teaspoons of celery juice three times a day, 1,000 mg of celery seed extract twice a day, or ½–1 teaspoon of celery oil (tincture) three times a day.

Design Your Own Diet

15. *Lycopene*—10 mg per day. You'll find lycopene in tomatoes and tomato products, guava, watermelon, apricots, pink grapefruit, and papaya.

16. *Supplements*—Take these vitamins, antioxidants, and nutraceutical supplements to round out the ideal diet:

Vitamin C	250–500 mg twice a day
Vitamin E	400–800 IU every day
Vitamin B_6	100 mg once or twice a day
Co-enzyme Q_{10}	60 mg once or twice a day
Lipoic acid	100–200 mg twice a day
N-acetyl cysteine	500 mg twice a day
L-arginine	2–3 grams twice a day
Hawthorn standardized extract	160–900 mg every day
L-carnitine	1,000 mg twice a day
Taurine	1.0–1.5 grams twice a day
Biotin	800 mcg twice a day

TRANSFORMING THE NUTRIENT LIST INTO REAL FOODS

Now let's look at some ways to convert the list above into a real-life eating plan.

Whenever possible, try to get your nutrients in the form of whole foods. Nutrients are better absorbed from whole foods, they're found in combination with other nutrients that help the body use them, and real foods taste better than pills.

Pump Up the Potassium

While restricting sodium is certainly an important part of the *Hypertension Institute Program*, increasing potassium may be almost as critical. As noted in Chapter 3, studies have repeatedly shown that people who consume a high-potassium diet or who take potassium supplements have lower blood pressure than those who take in low amounts of this mineral. Why? Because potassium acts like a natural diuretic, helping the body excrete excessive amounts of sodium, along with the fluid that sodium draws. Without enough potassium many people will retain water, which increases their blood volume and, in turn, pushes up their blood pressure.

Ironically, if you use diuretic medications to help ease water retention, you'll probably lose great quantities of potassium, the very mineral that guards against retaining water in the first place. Diuretics and corticosteroid drugs both leach potassium out of the body and wash it away in the urine. Your potassium stores can also be depleted through prolonged, heavy sweating, a high alcohol intake, overuse of laxatives, and/or frequent bouts of vomiting or diarrhea.

Because eating lots of potassium-rich foods can reduce the need for blood pressure medication in some people, I recommend that you eat at least six high-potassium foods every day. Luckily, high-potassium foods are easy to find and they taste good.

Foods Rich in Potassium

Food	Serving Size	Potassium (mg)
Apricots, dried	10 halves	482
Apricots, raw	3 medium	313
Avocado, California	½ medium	548
Avocado, Florida	½ medium	742
Banana	1 medium	451
Beans, green	3½ oz	260
Broccoli	1 cup	235
Cantaloupe	½ medium	812
Carrots	1 large	341
Chicken, white meat, without skin, roasted	½ breast	240
Dates	10	541
Flounder/Sole	3½ oz raw	366
Grapefruit, white	½ medium	175
Mushrooms	10 small	414
Orange	1 medium	250
Orange juice, fresh	½ cup	250
Peach	1 medium	171
Peanuts	1 oz	222
Pork, lean only, cooked	2 slices	311
Potato, baked	1 medium	503
Prunes	10	626
Raisins	⅓ cup	375
Salmon, raw	3½ oz	387
Spinach, cooked	½ cup	291
Squash, acorn, baked and mashed	½ cup	330
Sunflower seeds	¼ cup	210
Sweet potato, baked	1 small	300
Tomato	1 medium	254
Turkey, light meat without skin, roasted	3½ oz	305
Watermelon	1 cup	186

Maximize Your Magnesium

Studies of large populations have shown that the more magnesium people take in, the lower their blood pressures. This is partially due to magnesium's ability to relax the blood vessels, preventing constriction and spasm. Magnesium also helps to regulate the amount of sodium, calcium, and potassium found within the cells—three minerals that play key roles in maintaining healthy blood pressure levels.

You can find magnesium in a wide variety of foods, many of which are staples of the DASH diet. I recommend a magnesium intake of 500 to 1,000 mg per day, an amount you probably won't be able to get through food alone. So try to include at least two servings of the following magnesium-rich foods every day as a part of your DASH eating plan, then use supplements to make up the difference:

Good Sources of Magnesium

Food	Magnesium (mg)
Almonds, 1 oz	77
Avocado, Florida, ½ medium	52
Banana, 1 medium	33
Beans, butter, frozen, ½ cup	44
Beans, garbanzo, canned, ½ cup	80
Beans, lima, baby, frozen, ½ cup	46
Beet greens, ½ cup cooked	106
Bran flakes, ½ cup	35
Brazil nuts, 1 oz	64
Bread, whole wheat, 1 slice	26
Broccoli, raw, 2 stalks	48
Cashews, 1 oz	76
Cocoa powder, 1 tbsp	20

Design Your Own Diet

Cod, cooked, 3 oz	36
Collard greens, 3½ oz raw	57
Corn on the cob, 5½ inch ear	51
Halibut, broiled dry, 3 oz	90
Kale, raw, 3½ oz	37
Milk, nonfat, 1 cup	28
Noodles, egg, cooked, ½ cup	21
Oatmeal, cooked, 1 cup	56
Peanuts, 1 oz	59
Peas, dried, ¼ cup	81
Peas, green, frozen, ⅔ cup	25
Potato, raw, 1 medium	34
Rhubarb, frozen, raw, 1 cup	25
Shredded wheat, 1 biscuit	40
Shrimp, raw, 3 oz	30
Soybeans, 1 oz, dry	76
Spinach, raw, 3½ oz	88
Squash, summer, raw, ½ cup	16
Sunflower seeds, ¼ cup hulled	17
Tofu, 3½ oz	111
Tomato, raw, 1 large	28
Turnip greens, raw, 3½ oz	58
Wheat germ, 1 tbsp	37

Up Your Calcium Quotient

When your mother told you to drink your milk, she may have been doing your blood pressure, as well as your bones, a favor. Studies indicate that getting plenty of calcium may help reduce blood pressure and lower the risk of developing hypertension. On the DASH diet, two to three servings of dairy products are recommended, enough to give you about 850 mg of calcium. I strongly recommend that you consume all three servings and then use supplements to bring your intake up to the 1,000–1,500 mg range.

Some people might be tempted to skip the calories and just take supplements, but calcium is much better absorbed when it's in the form of food. So drink your milk!

Good Sources of Calcium

Food	Calcium (mg)
Yogurt, plain, nonfat, 1 cup	452
Milk, skim, l cup	302
Buttermilk, 1 cup	285
Swiss, 1 oz	272
Cheese, mozzarella, part-skim, 1 oz	207
Collard greens, frozen, chopped, ½ cup cooked	179
Ice milk, vanilla, 4 percent fat, 1 cup	176
Salmon, canned, with bones, 3 oz (low-sodium)	167
Sherbet, 2 percent fat, 1 cup	103
Kale, frozen, chopped, ½ cup cooked	90
Almonds, whole, 1 oz	75
Broccoli, frozen, chopped, ½ cup cooked	47

Zinc

Low levels of zinc have been linked to hypertension, coronary artery disease, Type II diabetes, and other ailments, which means that it's a good idea to get plentiful supplies of this mineral. I recommend 25 mg of zinc per day.

Good Sources of Zinc

Food	Zinc (mg)
Oysters, 6 medium	15.0
Beef shank, 3 oz lean only, cooked	8.9
Beef chuck, 3 oz lean only, cooked	7.4
Pork shoulder, 3 oz lean only, cooked	4.2
Breakfast cereal, 100 percent bran flakes, ¾ cup	3.7
Chicken leg, meat only	2.7
Yogurt, plain, 1 cup, low-fat	2.2
Cashews, dry roasted, 1 oz	1.6
Garbanzo beans, canned, ½ cup	1.3
Almonds, dry roasted, 1 oz	1.0

Parcel Out the Protein

Your protein intake should make up about 30 percent of your total calories. (An additional 40 percent of your calories should come from carbohydrates, and 30 percent from fat.) Non-animal sources of protein, such as beans, are preferable to animal sources such as hamburgers and steak. If you do eat animal protein, meat from lean or wild animals, such as range-fed cattle, is acceptable in moderation.

You should consume 1.0 to 1.2 grams of protein, per day, per kilogram of body weight. If you weigh 150 pounds, for example, you need 68 to 82 grams of protein per day, which is about the amount found in 6 ounces of meat plus 3 glasses of milk and 2 slices of bread.

You can also try these, either as part of your total protein intake, or as an addition:

Hydrolyzed whey protein	5 grams
Soy protein (fermented is best)	30 grams
Hydrolyzed wheat germ isolate	2–4 grams
Sardine muscle concentrate extra	3 mg

Don't Fill Up on Fats

Your total fat intake, including omega-3s, omega-6s, and omega-9s, should come to 30 percent of your total caloric intake. If you're consuming 2,000 calories per day, you should be taking in up to 700 of those calories in the form of fat (primarily the unsaturated kind).

We can break the fat component of the diet down even further:

- 10 percent of your fat intake, or 3–5 percent of your total caloric intake, should come from omega-3 PUFAs such as eicosapentaenoic acid (EPA) or docosahexaenoic acid (DHA) (e.g., fish oil).
- Another 50 percent of your fat intake, or 17.5 percent of your total caloric intake, should come from omega-9 MUFAs (e.g., olive oil).
- 10 percent of your total fat intake, or 3½ percent of your total caloric intake, should come from the omega-6 PUFAs (e.g., flaxseed oil, canola oil, or nuts).
- Less than 30 percent of your total fat intake should come from saturated fats.

Ten Percent Omega-3 PUFAs

The omega-3 fatty acids can do your cardiovascular system a world of good. Among other things, they help:

- reduce blood pressure
- quell inflammation
- reduce the tendency of platelets to stick together unnecessarily
- reduce fibrinogen (a blood-clotting protein)
- reduce irregular heartbeat (arrhythmia)
- reduce blood fat
- reduce atherosclerosis, coronary heart disease, and heart attacks

The best sources of omega-3s are cold-water fish and fish oils, although there are other good sources as well. I recommend an intake of 3 to 4 grams of omega-3 fatty acids per day. That translates to about:

- 1½ oz of cold-water fish rich in omega-3s (DHA and EPA); *or*
- 1–2 tsp of fish oil per day; *or*
- 3–5 3-oz servings of fish rich in omega-3 fatty acids per *week*

Cold-water fish that are good sources of omega-3s include:

- Anchovies
- Atlantic sturgeon
- Herring
- Mackerel
- Salmon
- Sardines
- Trout
- Tuna

Remember: If you eat your fish canned or otherwise preserved, be sure to get the low-sodium kind.

If you don't like fish or fish oil, you can boost your omega-3 levels in other ways:
- Take 1 tsp of flaxseed, canola, or fish oil daily.
- Eat whole grain products made with flax.
- Consider eating omega-3-enriched eggs, which come from hens fed diets containing ground flaxseed.[1] (Limit to 1 to 2 weekly.)
- Eat plenty of green leafy vegetables (such as broccoli, spinach, lettuce, greens).
- Get more legumes into your diet (pinto, navy, or lima beans; peas or split peas).
- Eat citrus fruit.

Fifty Percent Omega-9s

Omega-9s are monounsaturated fatty acids. The best known member of the omega-9 family is probably olive oil, which is proven to have a beneficial effect on both systolic and diastolic blood pressure.

For maximum results, I recommend a daily intake of 4 tablespoons of extra virgin olive oil. (Note: If you're on a weight loss diet, 4 tablespoons of oil will provide too many extra calories. Reduce your intake to 1 tablespoon daily.)

Ten Percent Omega-6 Fatty Acids

The omega-6 fatty acids can have indirect effects on hypertension. That is, they can prevent blood pressure increases caused by saturated fats, vasodilators, and stress.

Good sources of omega-6 fatty acids are:

- Flax, flaxseed, or flaxseed oil
- Canola oil
- Nuts
- Evening primrose oil
- Borage seed oil
- Black currant oil
- Conjugated linoleic acid (CLA)

I recommend a daily intake of 2 to 4 grams (about 1 teaspoon). If you're already taking a flaxseed product or canola oil to increase your omega-3s, don't double up on the dosage.

Lower Your Intake of Saturated Fats and Trans Fatty Acids

Most of the cholesterol that's manufactured in your body is made from the fat you eat, particularly saturated fat. Cholesterol then hitches a ride on a protein-based molecule called a lipoprotein. The high-density lipoprotein (HDL) molecule carries cholesterol out of the body, via the liver and intestines. But the low-density lipoprotein (LDL) molecule often deposits cholesterol on artery walls, where it can clog up the works and bring on atherosclerosis.

Saturated fat is particularly adept at driving up LDL levels, as is another kind of fat, the trans fatty acids. Trans fatty acids are polyunsaturated fats that have been artificially saturated with hydrogen. You've seen them listed on labels as "hydrogenated" fats, and they're found primarily in margarine, solid vegetable shortening, certain oils, store-bought baked goods, chips, microwave popcorn, some peanut butters, hot fudge topping, and some candies, to name a few. Many fast food chains cook their food in oil containing trans fatty acids.

To lower your LDL levels and help keep your artery walls

clean, it's important to decrease your intake of both saturated fat and trans fatty acids. Olive oil, which has been shown to help lower both cholesterol and blood pressure, should be used whenever possible instead of other kinds of fat. When the heavy taste of olive oil isn't appropriate, try canola oil, another monounsaturated fat that may help lower cholesterol.

Consider these suggestions for cutting back on saturated fat and trans fatty acids:

Instead of	Use
Milk, cheese, yogurt, or other dairy products made with whole milk, 2% or 1% fat	The fat-free version
Ice cream	Ice milk or frozen yogurt
Sour cream	Plain fat-free yogurt
Bottled, full-fat creamy salad dressing	Olive or canola oil and vinegar or lemon juice
Lard, meat fat, shortening	Olive or canola oil
Bologna or other luncheon meats	Sliced chicken or turkey (skinless) or lean roast beef
Butter or regular margarine	Fat-free margarine or low-fat mayonnaise
Heavily marbled meats (e.g., prime rib)	Lean cuts of beef (rump steak, flank steak, London broil) with all fat trimmed away
Poultry dark meat with skin	White meat with skin removed and all fat trimmed away before cooking
Vegetables in cream sauce or butter	Vegetables steamed, boiled, or baked without added fats, or stir-fried in a small amount of canola oil

Careful with the Carbohydrates

There's a great deal of controversy over carbohydrates these days, with some diet gurus proclaiming that all carbs are evil.

Part of the controversy stems from confusion as to what carbohydrates are, how they're used, and how they affect the body.

For the purposes of this discussion, we can think of two types of carbohydrates: simple carbohydrates and complex carbohydrates. There are several different kinds of simple carbohydrates, including maltose, lactose, glucose, fructose, galactose, and sucrose (table sugar). Simple carbohydrates are also known as refined carbohydrates or sugars. There are also different kinds of complex carbohydrates, including starches and dietary fibers.

We Americans eat plenty of carbohydrates, with a frightening amount in the form of the simple carbohydrates found in processed foods, white rice, processed wheat flour, sugary sodas, baked goods, sweetened canned foods, table sugar, and on and on. You can think of simple carbohydrates as the white foods—like white flour, white sugar, white rice, white bread. When you eat these simple carbohydrates, your bloodstream becomes flooded with glucose. To carry the glucose into your body's cells where it can be used for energy, the body produces the hormone insulin. But if you happen to be insulin-resistant, your body may need to produce quite a bit of this hormone in order to push that glucose into the cells. Unfortunately, excessive amounts of insulin floating through your bloodstream can damage the body. Complex carbohydrates don't inspire the flood of insulin that simple carbohydrates do, since they are broken down more slowly and their glucose is gradually released into the bloodstream. So although all carbs seem to have a bad name these days, it's the simple carbohydrates that are responsible for the lion's share of problems. Avoid or severely limit your intake of simple carbohydrates, while eating more of the complex kind, such as those found in broccoli, whole wheat flour, whole fruits and vegetables, and other similar foods.

Carbohydrates (primarily complex) should account for less than 40 percent of your total calories. In addition to fruits, vegetables, and whole grains, I recommend a daily intake of one of the following sources of complex carbohydrates:

Oatmeal	60 grams (2.1 ounces) per day
Oat bran (dry)	40 grams (1.4 ounces) per day
Beta glucan	3 grams (0.25 ounce) per day
Psyllium	7 grams (0.1 ounce) per day

Fire Up Your Fiber Intake

Dietary fiber is plant material that resists breakdown during the digestive process. There are two main kinds of fiber:

• *Insoluble fiber* is the woody or threadlike part of the shells and husks found in wheat bran, dried beans and legumes, or broccoli. It doesn't dissolve in water, so it speeds through the digestive system, bulking up the stool and sweeping toxic substances out of the body.

• *Soluble fiber* is found in the cell walls of certain grains, fruits, and vegetables. It does dissolve in water, forming a gel-like substance that helps sop up excess cholesterol in the digestive tract. Then the cholesterol is sent off for excretion, instead of being routed back into the bloodstream where it can clog up the arteries. The gel-like substance created by soluble fiber actually slows digestion (the opposite effect of insoluble fiber), but this is good for the body because it also slows the entrance of glucose into the bloodstream. So soluble fiber enhances blood sugar control and reduces insulin resistance.

Both kinds of fiber appear to help lower total cholesterol,

LDL ("bad") cholesterol and triglycerides, while increasing HDL ("good") cholesterol.

You'll find both types of fiber in just about all vegetables, fruits, and whole grains, but some good sources of each include:

Good Sources of Insoluble Fiber

Bananas
Broccoli
Brown rice
Brussels sprouts
Cauliflower
Corn
High-fiber cereal
Lentils
Potato (with skin)
Spinach
Wheat bran (unprocessed)
Whole wheat bread, pasta, crackers, or cereal

Good Sources of Soluble Fiber

Apples (particularly the skin)
Barley
Cabbage
Chickpeas
Flax seeds (ground seeds are best)
Lima beans
Nuts, most kinds
Oats, oatmeal, oat bran
Okra
Oranges, grapefruit

Pears (particularly the skin)
Pinto, navy, or kidney beans
Prunes
Psyllium seed
Split peas
Sweet potatoes

Water Warning!

You'll need to drink plenty of fluids when eating a high-fiber diet, or you may experience gastrointestinal problems like hard stools, constipation, gas, bloating, stomach aches, and, in extreme cases, intestinal blockages. Make sure you drink at least eight 8-ounce glasses of water daily, spread out throughout the course of the day.

Also, don't assume that since dietary fiber is good for blood pressure control, eating extra servings of high-fiber foods or taking spoonfuls of wheat bran is a great idea. Too much fiber can interfere with the absorption of important minerals, particularly calcium, iron, and zinc, and can bring on the gastrointestinal problems mentioned above. Instead, just stick to the recommended number of fruit, vegetable, and grain servings in the DASH diet. They should provide you with plenty of both kinds of fiber.

Other Helpful Foods

- *Garlic*—Eat 4 cloves or 4 grams of garlic per day. You can chop fresh garlic and add it to a stew or a stir-fry. You can also use it as a seasoning for vegetables, meat, poultry, fish, and soup.
- *Mushrooms*—Add shiitake and maitake mushrooms to your salads, or sauté them up as a side dish.

- *Guava fruit*—It's easy to enjoy this fruit; just slice it up and eat one or two per day.
- *Wakame seaweed*—This highly nutritious member of the brown algae family has been an important source of minerals in many Asian cultures for centuries. Rich in thiamin, niacin, vitamin C, iron, iodine, and calcium, it's used in soups, salads, vegetable dishes, and stir-frys. Buy it in its dried form and rehydrate in water before using. I recommend a daily intake of 3.0 to 3.5 grams of dried wakame seaweed, or about 2 tablespoons.
- *Celery*—Enjoy as a simple snack or an addition to your salad. I recommend that you eat plenty of this health-enhancing, nonfattening vegetable:

> 4 celery stalks per day
> *or* 8 teaspoons of celery juice three times a day
> *or* 1,000 mg of celery seed extract twice a day
> *or* ½ to 1 teaspoon of celery oil (tincture) three times a day

- *Lycopene*—This cousin of beta-carotene has antioxidant and other helpful properties. You'll find lycopene in tomatoes and tomato products such as pasta sauce, and in guava, watermelon, apricots, pink grapefruit, and papaya.

BLOOD PRESSURE ALERT: GO EASY ON CAFFEINE AND ALCOHOL!

Whether you follow the DASH diet or your own eating plan, there are two things you should either consume in moderation or avoid completely:

Cut Back on the Caffeine

There's controversy surrounding the caffeine question, but it's clear that caffeine is a stimulant, and a powerful one at that. A single cup of coffee drives up your blood pressure and heart rate and makes your arteries stiffer almost immediately, although these effects tend to be short-lived. Studies have shown that consumption of caffeine at a dose of about 2 cups of coffee for a 150-pound person drives up systolic blood pressure 5 to 9 mm Hg and diastolic pressure 3 to 8 mm Hg, if that person has been caffeine-free for twelve hours or more. Luckily, this effect subsides within about thirty to sixty minutes.[2] Similarly, people who consume 250 mg caffeine (about 2½ cups of drip coffee) three times a day for seven days can expect to see a significant increase in their diastolic blood pressure during the twenty-four hours after their first cup, but it subsides after a couple of days.[3]

Although most studies of large populations do not show a direct relationship between high blood pressure and caffeine intake,[4] it makes sense to stay away from anything that's going to drive your blood pressure up, even if it's only temporarily. With this in mind, try to keep your caffeine intake under 100 mg per day. And don't forget that many over-the-counter and prescription medications contain caffeine, sometimes quite a bit.

Design Your Own Diet

Common Sources of Caffeine

Coffee (6 oz cup)	Caffeine Content (mg)
Brewed	103
Instant	60
Decaffeinated	3

Tea (5 oz cup)	Caffeine Content (mg)
Black, 3 minute brew	42
Oolong, 3 minute brew	30
Instant dry powder, 1 tsp	32
Green, 3 minute brew	27

Soft drinks (12 oz)	Caffeine Content (mg)
Mountain Dew	54
Coca-Cola	45
Diet Coke	45
Tab	44
Dr. Pepper	40
Pepsi Cola	38
Diet Rite Cola	36

Chocolate and Cocoa	Caffeine Content (mg)
Baking chocolate (1 oz)	35
Sweet dark chocolate (1 oz)	20
Chocolate chips (¼ cup)	12
Cocoa powder, unsweetened (1 tbsp)	11
Cocoa beverage (6 oz, water mix)	10
Milk chocolate (1 oz)	6

Over-the-Counter Medications	Caffeine Per Standard Dose (mg)
Caffedrine (stimulant)	200
NoDoz (stimulant)	200
Vivarin (stimulant)	200
Aqua-Ban (diuretic)	200
Excedrin (pain relief)	130
Anacin (pain relief)	64
Midol (pain relief)	64

Prescription Medications	Caffeine Per Tablet or Capsule (mg)
Cafergot (migraine headaches)	100
Migralam (migraine headaches)	100
Norgesic Forte (muscle relaxant)	60
Esgic (sedative/analgesic)	40
Fiorinal (headaches)	40
Fioricet (headaches)	40
Darvon (pain relief)	32
Soma (pain relief/muscle relaxant)	32
Triaminicin (colds)	30

Watch Your Alcohol Intake

There's no doubt about it: Heavy consumption of alcoholic beverages drives up blood pressure[5] and is an important risk factor for stroke.[6] This is particularly true for chronic heavy drinkers. Initially, alcohol acts as a vasodilator (just think of the bloodshot eyes and ruddy complexion of a person who drinks a lot). But the body responds by clamping down on the blood vessels, so the end result of alcohol ingestion is vasoconstriction, which sends your blood pressure soaring.

Studies show that taking in more than 20 grams of alcohol per day (1½ to 2 drinks) increases both the risk and severity of hypertension. It also decreases the effectiveness of antihypertensive therapies by interfering with their action. The Atherosclerosis Risk in Communities study (ARIC) demonstrated that taking in any kind of alcoholic beverages in excess of 210 grams per week (about 16 beers) was an independent risk factor for hypertension.[7]

A heavy alcohol intake also interferes with your nutrient status. Alcohol provides no nutritional value; it's simply empty calories, which means that drinking too much of it can prompt weight gain. At the same time, alcohol dulls the appetite, so the more you drink the fewer nutritious foods you'll want to eat. Instead, you'll probably want to snack on high-sodium foods like chips and salted nuts—exactly what you don't need. And when you do eat some of the nutrient-dense foods that help control your blood pressure, alcohol can help block absorption of some key nutrients. Several vitamins and minerals are poorly absorbed due to alcohol ingestion, including magnesium and zinc, both of which are important for blood pressure control.

To make matters worse, alcohol stimulates the release of the hormone *cortisol*, which promotes both sodium retention and potassium loss. That, of course, pushes blood pressure up.

It's best if you avoid alcohol completely, but if you want to drink, do so in moderation. By that I mean less than 10 grams of alcohol per day, or the equivalent of:

- Less than 24 ounces of beer *or*
- Less than 10 ounces of wine (red wine is preferable, as it may have some heart-healthy benefits) *or*
- Less than 2 ounces of hard liquor

Remember also that many mixed drinks contain high amounts of sodium, sugar, and calories, so drinking limited amounts of straight beer, wine, or hard liquor may be a better idea, if you drink.

A FINAL REMINDER

This chapter listed foods and supplements for the do-it-yourself diet. It's separate from the VasoGuard Therapy and the DASH diet, and meant as an alternative. Either use the DASH diet and VasoGuard Therapy *or* your own diet plus the supplements listed in this chapter. Don't take the VasoGuard Therapy *and* the supplements, as they overlap, although you may add supplements that aren't included in the VasoGuard Therapy.

The idea is this:

1. The DASH diet gives you the basic eating plan that's been scientifically proven to lower blood pressure. In the DASH chapter, we also looked at a slimmed-down version of the modified DASH you can use if you need to lose weight. If you just follow the modified DASH, or the weight-loss DASH, you'll likely see vast improvements in your blood pressure, especially if you restrict your sodium intake.

2. My VasoGuard Therapy contains a short list of supplements I've found to be helpful in combating hypertension. The VasoGuard Therapy is *not* an alternative to the modified DASH diet; you should use both.

3. The lists of foods and supplements presented in this chapter give you an opportunity to create a do-it-yourself antihypertension diet.

Chapter 7

Prime the Pump with Exercise

Jim, a chubby, forty-two-year-old accountant for a large corporation, really liked his job, even though it involved a whole lot of sitting around. But being thirty-five pounds overweight with a blood pressure of 140/90 meant that a sedentary profession was the last thing he needed. When his doctor asked him about his exercise habits, Jim suddenly realized that practically all he ever did was shuffle from one chair to another. He'd get up in the morning, sit at the kitchen table to eat breakfast and read the paper, sit in his car for the long commute to work, park right by the elevator, walk about fifty steps from his car to his desk, and then sit there until lunchtime. Then he'd get in his car and drive to a restaurant, where he'd sit and eat lunch with a business associate, before driving back to work and sitting for the rest of the day. When he was through with work, he'd sit in his car for the drive home, then sit and eat his dinner and sit (or lie) on the couch until bedtime.

Jim started taking medication to control his blood pressure, but he was really motivated to get control of the problem himself so he could get off the drugs. With that in mind, he began a program of fast walking for one hour a day. Instead of driving to work, he commuted by train, which meant that he had to take a fifteen-minute walk to the station and another fifteen-minute walk to the office. Once he arrived, he walked up five flights of stairs to his office. Then, after he returned from lunch, he would walk up those stairs again before beginning his afternoon work. And at the day's end, it was another walk back to the station to get the train, and then the walk home. All in all, Jim spent one hour walking briskly, and about ten minutes walking up stairs. After one month, his doctor felt it was safe to discontinue his blood pressure medicine. And after two months, Jim's blood pressure was holding steady at 120/80, he'd dropped ten pounds, he had a lot more energy, and he felt like working even more exercise into his routine.

"I can't believe I didn't start an exercise program sooner," he said. "I haven't felt this good in years. It's by far the best thing I've done for myself in a long time!"

One of the most powerful nondrug remedies for the prevention and treatment of hypertension is exercise. Regular physical exercise can lower both systolic and diastolic blood pressure significantly. But don't worry, exercise doesn't mean endless hours at the gym. *You can effectively lower your blood pressure just by engaging in moderately intense physical activity,* such as brisk walking, for thirty to forty-five minutes a day, most days of the week.[1] A study that combined the results of thirteen other studies found that regular aerobic exercise brought about an average drop of 11.3 mm Hg in systolic blood pressure and 7.5 mm Hg in diastolic.[2]

This might sound strange: After all, exercise makes your heart beat harder and faster, and surely that must make your blood pressure rise, not fall! That's true: Your systolic blood pressure does rise while you're exercising, although your diastolic does not. But once you've finished your activity, your blood pressure will tend to drop to a level lower than before, and may stay at that level for several hours. A study of the short-term effects of physical activity on mildly hypertensive men found that the drop in their blood pressure lasted eight to twelve hours after they exercised, and their blood pressure was lower on exercise days than on inactive days.[3]

WHAT EXERCISE CAN DO FOR YOUR CARDIOVASCULAR SYSTEM

If I invented a pill that could drop your blood pressure significantly, lower your risk of having a heart attack or stroke, fight osteoporosis and Type II diabetes, help you lose weight and ease depression, make you look better and decrease your odds of dying, would you take it? Of course you would! Unfortunately, I don't have such a pill—but you can still get all of these results and more simply by exercising regularly. Regular exercise, performed just about every day, can:

• *Lower your blood pressure*—It can also significantly decrease your risk of developing hypertension in the first place.

• *Lower your LDL ("bad") cholesterol and total cholesterol*—High levels of either of these can clog up your arteries and contribute to coronary heart disease, heart attacks, and strokes. People who exercise can expect their total cholesterol to plummet by 24 percent and their LDL to fall by 10 percent, compared to their sedentary levels.[4]

• *Raise your HDL ("good") cholesterol*—Low levels of HDL, which carries cholesterol *away* from artery walls, are linked to a higher risk of coronary artery disease. Exercise raises HDL levels an average of 6 percent.[5]

• *Lower your triglycerides*—High levels of triglycerides (a type of blood fat) increase the risk of coronary artery disease.

• *Lower high blood glucose levels*—Too much glucose in the bloodstream (diabetes) can damage crucial organs, including the kidneys, heart, blood vessels, and eyes. Exercise helps improve insulin resistance, helping the body use glucose efficiently.

• *Improve endothelial function*—When the inner lining of the blood vessel malfunctions, blood vessels constrict and blood pressure rises. Exercise helps the blood vessels produce nitric oxide, a substance that makes them more elastic and better able to contract and relax efficiently. This results in improved blood flow and a decrease in blood pressure.

- *Reduce formation of dangerous blood clots*—Regular exercise helps reduce the clumping of blood platelets, which play an important role in the formation of dangerous blood clots that can trigger heart attacks and strokes.
- *Burn calories, reduce total body fat, help control weight*—Obesity puts an extra load on an already overworked heart and greatly contributes to hypertension.
- *Improve the blood flow to your coronary arteries*—Exercise helps the body feed the heart muscle itself.
- *Help manage stress*—Exercise helps burn off stress hormones, releases tension, and eases anxiety and depression, all of which can raise the blood pressure and put an extra burden on the heart.

Clearly, exercise is a crucial part of any program to combat hypertension. And not only does it help control hypertension, it lowers your risk of several potentially devastating diseases or conditions, including heart attacks, strokes, atherosclerosis, arteriosclerosis, diabetes, obesity, and osteoporosis. In fact, exercise reduces your overall risk of dying of *all* kinds of natural causes. The flip side, of course, is if you *don't* exercise, your inactivity is actually a risk factor for all of the above, especially hypertension. Researchers have found that sedentary people have a 20 to 50 percent increased risk of developing hypertension, as compared to more active, fit people.[6] And those who are very inactive are six times more likely to develop heart disease than those who are active.[7]

CAUTION: BEFORE BEGINNING OR CHANGING YOUR EXERCISE REGIMEN...

Don't start exercising, change your exercise, or increase the amount, intensity, or length of your exercises without first consulting your physician. It's important that everyone do so, and especially important if you have hypertension or any of its associated diseases.

WHAT KINDS OF EXERCISE SHOULD I DO?

To lower your blood pressure and improve your cardiovascular health, you'll need to get well acquainted with two kinds of exercise—aerobic and resistance.

• *Aerobic* means with oxygen, and aerobic exercises are those that increase both your intake of oxygen and your heart rate. Aerobic exercise is the prime method for conditioning your cardiovascular system. Just about any form of sustained movement that involves the large muscle groups can be considered aerobic exercise:

- bicycling
- walking
- swimming
- jogging
- dancing
- cross-country skiing
- rowing
- tennis
- vacuuming
- raking leaves
- digging in the garden
- mowing the grass (with a push mower)

Fast walking is usually the best exercise for beginners since it's familiar, there's no need for special equipment, the risk of injury is low, and just about anybody can do it. The key to aerobic exercise is to keep moving.

- *Resistance exercise* means working against some kind of force. That force may be weight (free weights, increasing the resistance on a stationary bike or rowing machine, and so on), gravity (the force you'll encounter when doing leg lifts), or water (which provides excellent resistance when you're swimming or doing water aerobics). Resistance training builds muscle strength and counters the atrophy brought on by aging, bed rest, or taking corticosteroids. It also burns fat, helps prevent osteoporosis, improves balance, and, when done properly, decreases the risk of future muscle injury. Finally, resistance exercise enhances your aerobic efforts by making you stronger, which increases your endurance. Resistance exercise usually involves the use of one or more of the following:
  - weight machines
  - free weights
  - cuff, hand, or ankle weights
  - the force of gravity (for example, leg lifts and chin-ups)
  - water (for example, water aerobics)
  - increasing the degree of incline or difficulty on a piece of exercise equipment, such as a stationary bicycle or rowing machine
  - elastic bands
  - wall pulleys

Even better is aerobic exercise *plus* resistance exercise. The combination of the two is the best prescription for cardiovascular fitness and all-around health. When planning your exercise program, pick two or three kinds of aerobic exercise, and two or three exercises that provide resistance. Then, mix them up for variety: Try cycling one day, brisk walking the next, and aerobic dancing on the third. You might rake leaves on another day or swim laps. The more diversity in your program, the more likely you'll be to enjoy your exercising and stick with it.

BECOMING MR. OR MS. FIT

Now that you know about aerobic and resistance exercise, you'll need to decide three important things: How often (*frequency*), how hard (*intensity*), and how long (*time*) you'll need to exercise to get maximum benefits. Frequency, intensity, and time are the keys to a successful exercise program. Put them all together and you get FIT!

Frequency

Don't worry—you're not going to have to live at the gym in order to do something about your hypertension. Studies have shown that even small amounts of exercise can help bring your blood pressure down. The most important thing is how often you're active, which leads me to the first rule of thumb when it comes to cardiac fitness:

Get into the habit of doing some kind of aerobic activity every day.

Out of the twenty-four hours that make up each day, there must be *one* little hour that you can devote to exercise. I strongly recommend that you engage in some kind of exercise every single day. Just taking a brisk, thirty-minute walk every day will lower your blood pressure somewhat, and most people can expect to see marked improvements after about eight to ten weeks. And if you increase the length and the intensity of these walks (up to a point), your blood pressure should drop even further. The second rule of thumb when it comes to cardiac fitness:

Resistance exercises should be done every day.

Both your resting blood pressure and your exercising pressure will be lower after training. And the strengthening of your skeletal muscles will make the effects even more pronounced. The best way to gain strength is to work against resistance, so you should perform a variety of muscle-resistance activities daily. Try doing lower extremity exercises (legs, abdominals, gluteals) one day, then upper extremity (arms, chest, and back) the next. It's best to work each muscle group two to three times a week. That way, you're not working every single muscle during every workout. This helps decrease your risk of overdoing it and injuring yourself, while still ensuring that you build strength and burn excess fat.

Be aware, however, that there are certain resistance exercises that can drive your blood pressure up, such as heavy weight lifting, isometric exercises, rope climbing, sit-ups, push-ups, shoveling snow, or anything that causes you to strain. Use light to medium weights; avoid bulking up and overdoing it. And if you feel that you're straining, ease off. The third rule of thumb when it comes to cardiac fitness:

Build some of your activity into your normal, everyday routine.

Slipping some extra exercise into the activities you'd be doing anyway—like shopping, housework, commuting to work—is a real time saver. That way, you can cut back on the length of your workouts yet still be sure to get in at least some exercise, no matter how hectic your day. If you ride your bike to work, for example, or park in the far corner of the parking lot and walk in, or take the stairs instead of the elevator, you may be able to cut back on the amount of time you spend at the gym later.

For maximum benefits, try to make each of your aerobic sessions last at least fifteen to twenty minutes, although *any* amount of exercise is beneficial. Even moderate and low-intensity activities have some long-term health benefits when they're done daily. So don't fall into the trap of saying to yourself, "I don't have time to do a whole exercise session today, so I'll just skip it." Even if you can only exercise for a minute, get to it!

Intensity

For an exercise to be truly aerobic, it must raise your heart rate to a certain level and keep it there through the active part of your workout. That certain level is called the *target heart rate zone*. So if you're not exercising hard enough to be in the zone, you're missing out on some of the cardioprotective effects of aerobic exercise. Coasting on your bicycle or strolling down the street doesn't cut it as aerobic exercise—you've got to get your heart beating faster and your breath coming harder. But it's also important that you don't exceed the target heart rate zone and put too much strain on your heart.

To figure out whether or not you're in the zone, first you'll need to learn to take your pulse:

1. Hold out one of your hands, palm side facing you. On the inner side of your wrist you'll notice a cordlike tendon running

straight down the middle. Using your opposite hand, put the tips of your index and middle fingers on top of that tendon, just below the point where the wrist meets the hand.

2. Then slide your fingertips toward the thumb side of your wrist until they come to rest in a little hollow right next to the tendon. This is a good place to feel your pulse.

3. Using a stopwatch or a clock with a second hand, count the number of pulse beats you feel during a 15-second interval.

4. Then multiply that number by 4 and you'll get the number of times your heart beats per minute (otherwise known as your heart rate).

Once you've warmed up and have been exercising for about ten minutes, take your pulse to determine your heart rate. If it's lower than the range indicated for your age group on the next page, you're probably not working hard enough. If it's higher, you need to slow down because you're doing too much.

TARGET HEART RATE ZONES

Look for your age in the left column of the table on the next page. Select the age closest to yours, then look at the corresponding numbers in the right-hand column. There you'll find two numbers separated by a dash. The lower number is 50 percent of the average maximum heart rate for your age; the higher number is 75 percent. You should keep your heart rate in this 50 to 75 percent range while doing your aerobic exercise. If you're just beginning an exercise program, try to keep your heart rate toward the lower end of the zone; if you're more fit, aim for the higher end of the zone.

Prime the Pump with Exercise

Age	Target Heart Rate Zone
20	100–150
25	98–146
30	95–142
35	93–138
40	90–135
45	88–131
50	85–127
55	83–123
60	80–120
65	78–116
70	75–113

As for resistance exercises, the intensity should be based on your current level of fitness. Ask your doctor which activities and what intensity levels are right for you. You may also want to consult a physical therapist or qualified trainer about how to start, and how to master the proper techniques. Supervised sessions are a good idea to make sure you're continuing to lift at the proper level and in the proper way. If you're overweight, older, or haven't exercised in a while, you'll need to start slowly and be careful that you don't overdo it.

Resistance training generally involves the strengthening of the muscles connected to each of the major joints—the shoulders, elbows, hips, knees, ankles, and feet. One exercise for each major muscle group could be a goal. Or, you can try doing more exercises while focusing on fewer muscle groups, then rotating to a different muscle group each day. The amount of weight or resistance you use will depend on what your body can handle. It's best to start with what feels easy to you, then gradually add weight or resistance over time. When trying a new exercise, use no weight or resistance at all until you get the hang of it. Then try it with a one-pound weight or some slight resistance. Don't be in too much of a rush to add more weight. Listen to your body and to your physical therapist or trainer. The last thing you want to do is strain your muscles or your heart.

A good general goal may be something like: 12 to 15 lifts (or to muscle fatigue) of a light to medium weight equal one set. Do three sets per session.

Time

You need to get some aerobic and some resistance exercise just about every day, and you should exercise intensely enough to reach but not exceed your target heart rate zone. But how long do you need to exercise each day? Is ten minutes enough? Is an hour too much? One way to tell, believe it or not, is through the amount of calories you burn.

Burn Those Calories!

The Harvard Alumni Health Study[8] found that burning at least 2,100 calories per week through exercise decreased the risk of coronary heart disease. But burning more than 2,100 calories a week was even better. Men who burned 2,100 to 4,199 calories weekly through exercise reduced their risk of coronary heart disease by 10 percent, but those who burned 4,200 calories or more reduced their risk 19 percent—almost twice as much. However, the reduced risk plateaued at 4,200 calories. That is, those who burned more than 4,200 calories didn't decrease their risk of coronary heart disease any more than 19 percent.

Burning 4,200 calories per week, then, is our goal for maximal heart protective effect. What does that translate into exercise? Take a look at the following chart. It gives the *approximate* amount of calories burned during various activities by a 150-pound person who is exercising within the target heart rate zone. (This chart is just meant to give you a *rough* idea of calorie expenditure. The amount of calories you actually burn will depend on your weight, your muscle mass, the speed of your metabolism, how fit you are, and the intensity of your workout.)

Kind of Exercise	Calorie Expenditure	
	30 minutes	60 minutes
Aerobic exercise, land	340	685
Aerobic exercise, water	145	280
Bicycling—12 mph	280	565
Bicycling—18 mph	430	850
Cleaning house	120	210
Cross-country skiing	300	585
Floor washing	180	350
Jogging, 1 mile/10 minutes	365	730
Jumping rope	285	575
Lawn mowing, manual	140	250
Racquetball	230	455
Rowing machine	210	410
Stair climbing	310	600
Swimming, 50 yards/minute	260	525
Tennis, singles	235	465
Vacuuming	135	250
Walking, 1 mile/20 minutes, flat	120	240
Walking, 1 mile/20 minutes, hill	165	325

An Hour a Day!

Using this chart as a guide, you can see that it would take about an hour a day of moderate to intense aerobic exercise to burn 4,200 calories a week. You could probably still meet this goal with about forty-five minutes of moderately intense aerobic exercise, plus about fifteen minutes of resistance training every day.

Now, don't throw in the towel because it sounds like way too much time and effort. Start by taking a brisk thirty-minute walk every day. If you feel fine doing that, make it two brisk walks—one in the morning, one in the evening (or on your lunch hour). If you carry a one- to two-pound weight in each hand and swing your arms, you'll be getting some upper body resistance work done at the same time. There—you've just established a one-hour-a-day exercise habit! As you become stronger and more comfortable with exercising, you will want to branch out into other activities and put together some sort of resistance training program for yourself. But in the beginning, just walk!

Break It Up

It's okay to break your one-hour exercise session up into smaller sessions. Just remember that for aerobic benefits, you'll need to exercise within your target heart rate zone for thirty to forty-five minutes at a time. For resistance training, you should do the full number of reps for a given muscle group all at once.

And don't forget: Your exercise session should always include some kind of warm-up and cool-down to prevent muscle injury, gradually increase your heart rate, and then ease it back down to normal at the session's end.

Do the Combo Thing

Some exercises provide both aerobic benefits and resistance training, like cycling on an incline, walking uphill or with ankle weights, cross-country skiing, swimming, water aerobics, or rowing, among others. If you do these or similar exercises, you may be able to cut back on the length of your session, since the forty-five minutes of aerobics can also qualify as a full session of resistance exercise. But few exercises will strengthen all of your muscle groups, so you'll probably need to spend at least some time working on resistance exercises alone.

DECIDE TO DO IT

The hardest part about exercising, I believe, is making the commitment to do it. Once you do, everything will fall into place. You *do* have the time and the opportunity to exercise—you just have to make it a top priority. A lot of people like to exercise first thing in the morning for this very reason. They make sure they get their exercise session in before other things come up to throw them off track. It also helps to pick fun activities that you'll enjoy doing. If you love your aerobic dance class or playing tennis with a friend, build it into your exercise schedule. Then you'll be having fun and working on your fitness at the same time. How about jazz dancing? A good, active jazz dance class can rev up your heart, strengthen your lungs, and increase muscle tone body-wide—all at the same time.

THE ULTIMATE EXERCISE PRESCRIPTION FOR LOWERING YOUR BLOOD PRESSURE

In the best of all worlds, I would recommend the following exercise prescription for my hypertension patients:

- 45 minutes of daily aerobic exercise
- Resistance exercises daily, or at least 3 times a week, rotating the workout so that each muscle group is exercised 3 times a week
- Burn 4,200 calories per week through exercise

Put into a weekly schedule, the Ultimate Exercise Prescription might look something like this:

The Ultimate

Monday
Aerobic: Bicycling—18 mph (30 minutes)
Lawn mowing—manual (15 minutes)
Resistance: Weights: Upper body—back, chest, shoulders, triceps, biceps

Tuesday
Aerobic: Brisk walking (45 minutes)
Resistance: Weights: Lower body—Abdominals, gluteals, quadriceps, hamstrings, calves

Wednesday
Aerobic: Aerobic exercise, land (45 minutes)
Resistance: Swimming, 50 yards/minute (15 minutes)

Thursday
- *Aerobic:* Bicycling—18 mph (30 minutes)
- *Resistance:* Weights: Upper body—back, chest, shoulders, triceps, biceps

Friday
- *Aerobic:* Stair climbing (30 minutes)
- *Resistance:* Rowing machine (15 minutes)

Saturday
- *Aerobic:* Aerobic exercises, water (45 minutes)
- *Resistance:* Weights: Lower body—abdominals, gluteals, quadriceps, hamstrings, calves

Sunday
- *Aerobic:* Tennis singles (45 minutes)
- *Resistance:* Swimming, 50 yards/minute (15 minutes)

The Lite Version

But let's say you're more of a beginner and you need to do lighter exercise that fits into your life more easily. How about this?

Monday
- *Aerobic:* Brisk walk around neighborhood, flat (15 minutes) (A.M.)
  Brisk walk around neighborhood, hill (15 minutes) (P.M.)
- *Aerobic/Resistance:* Vacuuming (15 minutes)

Tuesday
Aerobic: Brisk walk around neighborhood, flat (15 minutes) (A.M.)
Aerobic/ Resistance: Stationary bicycle—incline setting (30 minutes) (P.M.)

Wednesday
Aerobic/ Resistance: Water aerobics class (1 hour)

Thursday
Aerobic: Rake leaves (30 minutes)
Resistance: Wash floors (30 minutes)

Friday
Aerobic: Climb the stairs at work (do 15 minutes' worth of climbing, even if you have to come back down and climb up again)
Aerobic/ Resistance: Brisk walk around neighborhood, including some up hill walking (30 minutes)
Resistance: Do upper body exercises with free weights (15 minutes)

Saturday
Aerobic: Go out dancing! (Remember to keep moving; don't sit on the sidelines) (45 minutes continuous)
Resistance: Rent a canoe and paddle (15 minutes)

Sunday
Aerobic: Take a hike in the mountains on a trail that inclines (45 minutes)

Resistance: Hold a 1-2 lb free weight in each hand as you hike, and swing your arms (15 min) (you can carry them in your backpack after that)

If this still looks like too much, just start by walking every day. The important thing is to get moving, and keep moving regularly!

CAUTION!

If you have any of these symptoms while exercising, you're doing too much. Stop immediately and see your health care practitioner if symptoms persist or are severe:

- Blurred vision
- Chest pain
- Cold chills
- Dizziness
- Excessive shortness of breath
- Extreme fatigue
- Fainting
- Headache
- Light-headedness
- Nausea
- Vomiting

TEN TIPS TO HELP YOU MAKE YOUR EXERCISE PROGRAM A SUCCESS

1. Before beginning any exercise program, see your doctor for a thorough medical evaluation, and to determine the kinds and amounts of exercise that are right for you.

2. Realize that you're going to feel a little tired during your exercise sessions and a little stiff or sore during the next day or two. Both are normal. Remember that you need to put a certain amount of stress and strain on your body in order to increase strength and endurance. If you only do what's easy and comfortable, you won't improve. But sometimes it's a fine line that separates enough from too much. Err on the side of caution. If your body says no, listen to it.

3. Don't overdo it. Doing too much too soon can lead to health problems, injuries, or burnout. Start slowly and increase the length and/or intensity of your workouts gradually, as you gain strength and endurance.

4. Be consistent. You need to get some kind of exercise every day. We've all heard of the Weekend Warrior who does nothing Monday through Friday, then tries to run a marathon on the weekend. This is a great way to injure yourself or bring on a major cardiovascular accident (that is, a heart attack or stroke). The quantity of exercise you get is less important than consistency and frequency.

5. Breathe. Exercise greatly increases the amount of oxygen your body needs, so breathe deeply and rhythmically throughout your session. Holding your breath can drive your blood pressure up and contribute to excessive muscle soreness.

6. Pick fun activities. If you feel that exercise is drudgery, you're probably not going to stick with it. Do things you enjoy; exercise with a friend; add music.

7. Include some variety in your exercise program. Walking is great, but if you're doing it seven days a week it might get boring. Mix up your activities so you have something different to look forward to.

8. Wear comfortable clothes and shoes. Wear loose-fitting clothing that doesn't hinder movement—but make sure it's not so loose that it might catch in your bicycle chain, weight machine, or anything else. Your clothing should be made of lightweight fabrics that breathe, letting air in and moisture out. And it's a must that you get a good pair of supportive shoes that don't pinch or rub.

9. Always warm up and cool down. Get your body into the exercise mode gradually by walking at a moderate pace, doing gentle jumping jacks, or slowly jogging in place for a few minutes before you start your activity. Generally, you can consider yourself warmed up when you've broken a sweat. Then, when you've finished your exercise or activity, don't stop abruptly. Ease your body back down to normal, ending your session with some moderate or slow walking until your heart rate decreases and you no longer have to huff and puff. This is a great time to do some stretching, as your muscles will be nice and warm, making it less likely that you'll injure them.

10. Drink plenty of water. You can't rely on thirst to let you know when you need to rehydrate. By the time you're thirsty, dehydration may have already set in. Drink a glass of water before exercising, and bring along a bottle of water to sip from throughout your session. Then drink another glass or two after you've finished.

ON YOUR MARK, GET SET . . .

Run, swim, dance, garden, vacuum, hit a ball, kick a ball, dance to the music—it doesn't matter what you do, as long as it keeps your heart beating in the target zone for fifteen minutes or more or strengthens your muscles—or does both.

My prescription for exercise is simple: See your physician to discuss the best exercises for you, and then do it. No matter how modest your program is to begin with, get started!

Chapter 8

De-Stress Your Life

Stress does more than ruin your mood. Mental stress makes your nervous system leap into action, with potentially harmful results. You've experienced this many times: Just think of how your body would react if you were suddenly asked to stand up and deliver an impromptu speech to a large group. There's a good chance your heart would start to pound and you'd begin to perspire. Perhaps your breathing would become shallow and rapid, and your face might get hot while your hands grow icy. If someone were to take your blood pressure right then and there, it would undoubtedly be higher than it normally is. That's because the sympathetic nervous system's normal response to stress includes increases in heart rate, vascular resistance, the thickness of the blood, and the stickiness of the blood platelets—all of which jack up the blood pressure.

When you're stressed, your body prepares itself to handle a *physical* emergency, even if the stress is 100 percent mental. Your bloodstream is flooded with supercharged stress hormones like adrenaline, norepinephrine, and cortisol, giving you the strength and energy to physically fight off an enemy or run for your life—or both. All of this is very helpful when a mugger is chasing you down an alley, or if you need to lift a two-ton car all by yourself in order to free a loved one trapped beneath it. In cases like these, the stress response is a lifesaver.

But what if there's no physical outlet for your stress response. Suppose you're furious with your boss but have to hold your tongue. Or maybe your stress response is triggered over and over as you battle difficult customers, traffic, family problems, and so on. In either case, the results can be extremely hard on your body and your health. Just imagine the superstressed person facing the equivalent of emergency after emergency, day after day, heart pumping like crazy, blood vessels constricting, blood platelets ready to clump together, and blood pressure skyrocketing. Something similar happens in the case of the hot reactor. These people have exaggerated sympathetic responses to everyday stresses, even small ones. They might not actually have more stress in their lives than anyone else, but for them, getting cut off in traffic has the same internal effect as meeting a grizzly bear in the woods. Since every little stressor sends their bodies into overdrive, it's not surprising that hot reactors often develop atherosclerosis and chronic hypertension.

Any way you cut it, excessive amounts of stress are bad for your body—and the effects on your blood vessels are particularly devastating. Repeated stimuli from the sympathetic nervous system injures the all-important endothelium, the inner lining of the arteries. This, in turn, makes the blood vessels tighten up and become more prone to developing atherosclerosis. Unfortunately, atherosclerotic blood vessels become even more constricted in response to sympathetic stimuli. So the more you're stressed, the more your blood vessels clamp down and the more your blood pressure rises. After a while, your blood vessels no longer know how to relax, and your hypertension may become chronic.

It doesn't require a terrible mental stress to make your arteries tighten up. Routine activities, such as hearing a loud noise, accidentally breaking a glass, or having a chat with your boss can raise your systolic blood pressure 5 to 10 mm Hg, or more. Even brief periods of mental stress can cause temporary endothelial dysfunction *in healthy people* for as long as four hours after the event.[1]

However, it's chronic stress that really takes a toll on the body and contributes heavily to hypertension. The stress of working long hours, for example, can significantly increase your risk of hypertension, heart attacks, and diabetes mellitus. If you've got a job that's demanding but allows you very little control (think of Lucy and Ethel in the chocolate factory), there's a good chance that both your blood pressure and blood fats will rise. To make matters worse, people who have too much stress in their lives often compensate by developing unhealthy habits like smoking, drinking, or overeating, all of which can contribute to hypertension.

ISN'T PHYSICAL STRESS ALSO DANGEROUS?

Studies have shown that mental stress can be much more damaging to the body than the routine physical stresses we encounter while going about our normal daily activities or exercising properly. One such study[2] looked at 196 patients, ages forty to seventy-five, who had stable coronary artery disease. The researchers tested the volunteers' physiological reactions to mental stress (via public speaking and a color-word test) as opposed to physical stress (via a stationary bike). When the patients were told to pretend they had been caught shoplifting and had to prepare and deliver a three-minute defense in front of a group, their vascular resistance increased markedly. But when they rode stationary bikes with the workload increased at regular intervals, their vascular resistance decreased. This is most likely because the mental stress triggered the release of epinephrine (adrenaline), which causes vasoconstriction. But the stationary bike challenge didn't alter epinephrine levels, so the blood vessels were able to relax and deliver a greater supply of blood to the working muscles, as they should.

HOW DO YOU KNOW IF YOU'RE STRESSED?

We're all hit with a certain amount of stress in our lives. Some of us can handle it fairly well, even large amounts. But at some point you'll find yourself on overload, stretched to the breaking point, up to your eyebrows, and just plain stressed out. For the sake of your physical, mental, and emotional health, it's best to recognize the symptoms of impending stress overload before you actually get to the end of your rope. Then you can scale back your responsibilities and activities and take things a little easier. If you should find yourself exhibiting one or more of these symptoms, you probably need to find more effective ways to manage and release your stress:

- alcohol abuse
- anxiety
- apathy
- back aches
- chronic anger
- clenching of the jaw

- crying excessively
- depression
- drug abuse or dependency
- edginess
- fatigue
- headaches
- heart palpitations
- insomnia
- light-headedness
- loneliness
- overeating
- racing heart
- stomach aches
- sweaty palms
- tightness in the shoulders or neck
- teeth grinding

ANXIETY, DEPRESSION, AND LONELINESS

Mental stress often manifests as anxiety or depression, or sometimes both—and each increases the risk of developing hypertension. One study gathered data from nearly 3,000 people, ages twenty-five to sixty, who participated in the National Health and Nutrition Examination Survey (NHANES), a long-range study that has been following some 14,000 Americans since 1975. All of the volunteers for the anxiety/depression study had normal blood pressure in the beginning. They had their blood pressures taken and they filled out a questionnaire that evaluated symptoms of anxiety and depression. Ten years later, the subjects had their blood pressure readings taken again. Those who had scored high in either anxiety or depression on the initial questionnaire had two to three times the risk of developing hypertension during the next ten years. In whites, the risk doubled only after the age of forty-five, but in African-Americans, the risk tripled and was seen in all age groups.[3]

Stress in the form of loneliness can also push up blood pressure. One study of older people, ages sixty-five to seventy-eight, found that those who were lonely had blood pressures an average of 16 points higher than those who were not lonely.[4]

THE GOOD NEWS

It's impossible to avoid all of the stressors of life, but you can do something to lessen their effects on your physical, mental, and emotional health. One antidote to the stress response is the *relaxation response*, which takes you to a deep state of restfulness while you remain awake. Dr. Herbert Benson, founder of the Mind/Body Medical Institute at Harvard Medical School, developed the relaxation response as a way to reverse stress-induced damage to the body. The response taps into an area of your brain that releases and diminishes your physical responses to stress. When practiced regularly, the relaxation response can effectively slow your metabolism, decrease your heart rate and muscular tension, and lower your blood pressure. By experiencing deep relaxation for just twenty minutes a day, you can do a lot to relieve your stress and bring your blood pressure down to a more healthful level.

The relaxation response, also called *progressive relaxation*, is easy to do, takes no equipment, and feels great. Just find a quiet, comfortable place where you can be alone for twenty minutes and follow these steps:

• Sit in a comfortable chair or lie on a mat on the floor and close your eyes.

- If you're lying down, let your arms lie at your sides. If you're sitting, let your hands lie relaxed in your lap.
- Take a deep breath: Slowly inhale for 4 counts, hold for 4 counts, and exhale for 4 counts. Repeat, if desired, then resume breathing normally.
- Focus on your feet: Relax them completely, letting all the tension go, until they feel so heavy and relaxed that you can hardly imagine moving them.
- Then focus on your ankles and repeat the process.
- Gradually work your way up through your body, relaxing all of your muscles, one by one, including those in your face and head.
- Take the entire 20 minutes to complete the process. When you're finished, gradually begin to wake up again by wiggling your fingers and toes, and gently shaking out your arms and legs. You may also want to do some easy stretching.
- Take your time getting up, especially if you've been lying down. Slowly and gently ease yourself back into the real world.

A BETTER APPROACH TO SMOOTHING DOWN STRESS?

Although progressive relaxation is an excellent tool for physically relaxing the body and lowering the blood pressure, a mental form of relaxation called Transcendental Meditation (or TM) may be even better. The Indian yogi Maharishi Mahesh first introduced TM to the Western world back in the 1960s. Now in use by over four million people worldwide, its effectiveness as a stress reliever is beginning to be accepted by even the most traditional medical establishments.

In 1995, researchers pitted TM (the mental approach to relaxation) against progressive relaxation (the physical approach) to see which was most effective at lowering blood pressure. One hundred twenty-seven mildly hypertensive African-Americans between the ages of fifty-five and eighty-five took part in the study. Progressive relaxation worked well: It lowered systolic blood pressure an average of 4.7 mm Hg and diastolic 3.3 mm Hg. But TM proved to be the big winner, lowering systolic blood pressure by 10.7 mm Hg and diastolic by 4.7 mm Hg. As an antihypertensive technique, TM proved to be about twice as effective as progressive muscle relaxation.[5] TM is also associated with a lessening of atherosclerosis, lowered cholesterol, and a decrease in rates of hospitalization.[6] (For unknown reasons, other forms of meditation haven't produced such beneficial results.) More and more, doctors are beginning to realize the value of Transcendental Meditation as a method for preventing and treating coronary heart disease.

TM is easy to learn, but it takes practice to be able to do it right. The more you do it, however, the easier it will become. But first you'll need to decide on a word or short phrase (such as "love" or "universe" or "we are one") that you'll feel comfortable repeating to yourself silently, over and over again. If you take private instruction in TM, you'll be given a word (a mantra) to repeat. Either way, the silent repetition of a word or phrase will induce deep relaxation. Once you've got your word or phrase, follow these steps:

• Find a place where you can sit quietly in a comfortable position and close your eyes.

• Inhale and exhale slowly but naturally as you silently repeat your word or phrase. Concentrate solely on your word or phrase as you try to keep your mind completely blank.

• As thoughts and feelings come into your mind, simply let them go and return your concentration to your word or phrase.

Stay relaxed; don't get anxious about these stray thoughts. Just acknowledge that they are there and dismiss them.
- Continue your repetition for 10 to 20 minutes, then slowly open your eyes.
- Gently and gradually ease yourself back into the conscious world before standing up and going on your way.
- Repeat twice a day.

OTHER STRESS BUSTERS

Of course, TM and progressive relaxation aren't the only ways to relieve and manage the stress in your life. Exercise is a key element in stress relief. Deep breathing, yoga, t'ai chi, qigong, self-hypnosis, aromatherapy, warm baths, prayer, relaxation tapes, and soothing music are all effective ways of bringing your blood pressure, heart rate, muscle tension, and breathing down to lower, more healthful levels. As with any health practice, the one that works the best is the one you'll do regularly. And the one you'll do regularly is undoubtedly the one you like the best. So take your pick! Or mix and match. Just do some form of stress-relieving activity at least twenty minutes every day.

Stress is here to stay. Difficult customers, demanding bosses, terrible traffic, government scandals, and all the rest aren't going away. But what can change is your reaction to the inevitable annoyances and disasters of life. You can learn to turn off your overreaction to stress, and blunt its ability to send your blood pressure soaring.

Chapter 9

If Medicine Is Necessary

In an ideal world, the combination of diet, exercise, and the other lifestyle modifications we've talked about would, by themselves, pull your elevated blood pressure right back down to a safe level. And while that does happen in many cases, it doesn't always. Some people have alarmingly high pressure that must be reduced by drugs. Others find it too difficult to change their ways. Whatever the reason, antihypertensive medications continue to be necessary for many people and, if prescribed wisely and used properly, they're very effective.

Taking medication to reduce your elevated blood pressure will automatically reduce your risk of cardiovascular disease and death. In fact, studies have shown that antihypertensive medications not only fight hypertension, but also help prevent strokes, heart attacks, heart failure, exacerbation of kidney disease, and death from all causes in hypertensives. The elderly enjoy an even more pronounced drop in the risk of coronary heart disease when their hypertension is treated.[1] And many studies have shown that reducing elevated blood pressure can help just about everyone, no matter how high their pressure was to begin with, no matter their age, race, sex, or socioeconomic status. This means that millions of people can rest easy, knowing that their health is being enhanced and their lives extended through the use of antihypertensive medicines.

Unfortunately, most medications have side effects—some slight, some heavy-duty—and they usually involve at least some out-of-pocket costs.

In this chapter, we'll look at how doctors decide whether or not to prescribe antihypertensive medicines; the classes of medicines they use; the selection process; what you can expect them to do for you and what to watch out for.

WHEN TO BRING OUT THE PRESCRIPTION PAD

To prescribe or not to prescribe: That's a key question for your physician, who knows that the right dosage of the right medicine at the right time for the right patient can truly be a lifesaver. But the wrong medicine may be more than a waste of time and money, as it can trigger potentially dangerous side effects such as heart palpitations and dizziness.

Because of this, the Joint National Committee on Prevention, Detection, Evaluation, and Treatment of High Blood Pressure[2] has developed guidelines to help doctors determine, among other things, who really needs to take antihypertensive medication. Using the guidelines, the first thing your doctor will do is determine whether you have any of these major risk factors:

- Over the age of sixty
- Male
- Postmenopausal woman

- Family history of cardiovascular disease *and* being a male older than fifty-five or a female older than sixty-five
- Smoker
- Dyslipidemia (elevated cholesterol and blood fats)
- Diabetes mellitus

Then your doctor will determine whether you've suffered any hypertension-related organ damage (target organ disease) or if you have any signs of cardiovascular disease. He or she will take a thorough medical history and perform a physical exam to find out whether you currently have, or have had, any of the following:

- Heart disease (left-ventricular hypertrophy, angina, a heart attack in the past, prior coronary revascularization, or heart failure)
- Stroke
- Transient ischemic attack ("baby stroke")
- Kidney disease (nephropathy)
- Peripheral artery disease (such as atherosclerosis)
- Retinopathy

Finally, your doctor will compare your risk factors and target organ damage to your blood pressure to see if medicines are called for. The chart[3] on the facing page makes it easy.

TYPES OF ANTIHYPERTENSIVE MEDICATIONS

If your physician decides that you do need to take medication for your hypertension, he or she will have to choose from numerous antihypertension medications. These drugs fall into several categories (text continued on page 190):

Algorithm for treatment of hypertension

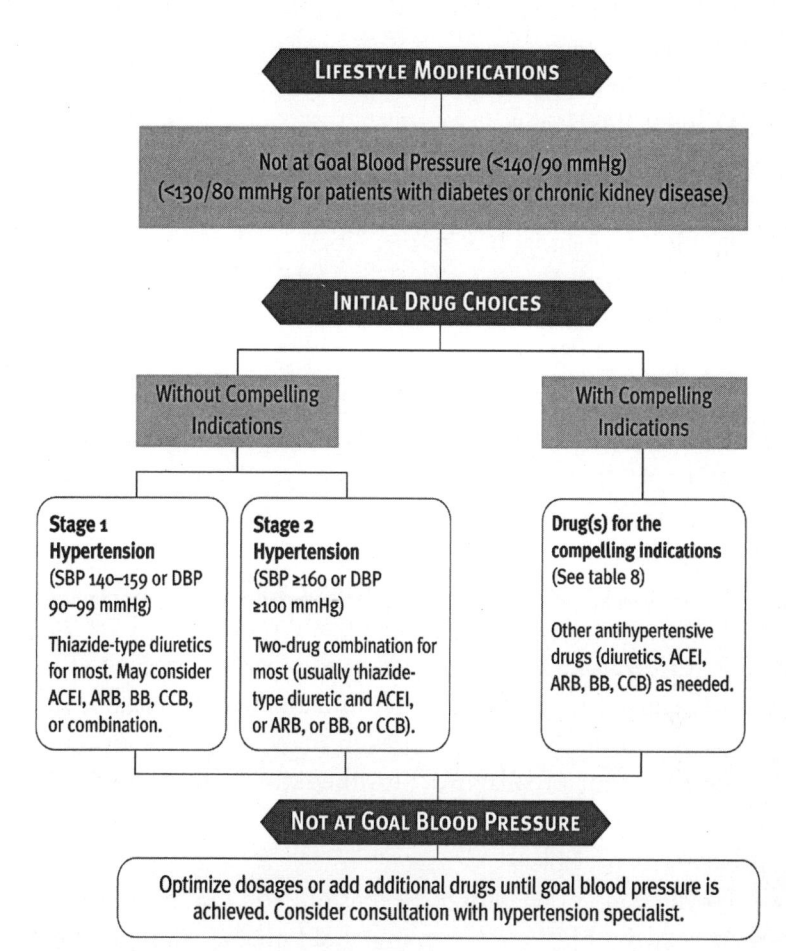

LIFESTYLE MODIFICATIONS

Not at Goal Blood Pressure (<140/90 mmHg)
(<130/80 mmHg for patients with diabetes or chronic kidney disease)

INITIAL DRUG CHOICES

Without Compelling Indications

Stage 1 Hypertension
(SBP 140–159 or DBP 90–99 mmHg)

Thiazide-type diuretics for most. May consider ACEI, ARB, BB, CCB, or combination.

Stage 2 Hypertension
(SBP ≥160 or DBP ≥100 mmHg)

Two-drug combination for most (usually thiazide-type diuretic and ACEI, or ARB, or BB, or CCB).

With Compelling Indications

Drug(s) for the compelling indications
(See table 8)

Other antihypertensive drugs (diuretics, ACEI, ARB, BB, CCB) as needed.

NOT AT GOAL BLOOD PRESSURE

Optimize dosages or add additional drugs until goal blood pressure is achieved. Consider consultation with hypertension specialist.

DBP, diastolic blood pressure; SBP, systolic blood pressure.

Drug abbreviations: ACEI, angiotensin converting enzyme inhibitor; ARB, angiotensin receptor blocker; BB, beta-blocker; CCB, calcium channel blocker.

- diuretics
- central alpha agonists
- beta blockers
- direct vasodilators
- alpha$_1$-blockers
- combined alpha-beta blockers
- ACE inhibitors (ACEIs)
- calcium channel blockers (CCBs)
- angiotensin II receptor blockers (ARBs)
- postganglionic neuron inhibitors

Why so many types of drugs? Hypertension is a multifaceted disease with many causes and consequences, which means it can be attacked in several different ways. Suppose, for example, you were a general about to go into battle against a fierce and terrible enemy. You could send your army out to meet the enemy head-to-head on the battlefield and try to crush him with brute strength alone. Or, you could try to cut off his supplies. You could also bomb some of the roads he needs to use, so only part of his army could get into action. Then again, you could bomb the factories he uses to make his tanks and guns so he'd run out of weapons. In other words, there are many ways to fight a war and a wise general will use as many approaches as possible.

It's the same thing with hypertension. You can try to destroy the enemy by breaking his stranglehold on the arteries, taking away some of the blood volume he uses to keep the pressure up, interfering with his ability to manufacture "weapons" like angiotensin-II, preventing his "messengers" from delivering their dispatches, and so on. Medications can accomplish all of these tasks. In a sense:

If Medicine Is Necessary

- Diuretics destroy one of the enemy's main "weapons"—excess fluid in the body—and dilate arteries.
- Beta blockers interfere with the enemy's "manufacturing procedures," preventing him from converting harmless substances into angiotensin-II, which raises blood pressure.
- Calcium channel blockers prevent too many "enemy soldiers" (calcium) from infiltrating into the arterial smooth muscle and causing contraction.
- Central alpha agonists take away one of the enemy's "weapons" by reducing the amount of adrenaline.
- Alpha blockers interfere with the enemy's "communications" by blocking their access to vital receptor sites.

Your doctor can take a one-drug approach to combating hypertension; that's called monotherapy. Or he or she can use two or more types of drugs, attacking hypertension in several ways at once. When deciding which drug or drugs to prescribe, your physician may follow these guidelines set forth by the Joint National Committee on Prevention, Detection, Evaluation, and Treatment of High Blood Pressure:

- Begin with a low dose of a selected drug (or combination).
- Slowly increase the dose, if necessary, according to the patient's needs, responses to the drug, and age.
- Ideally, the patient should only have to take the drug(s) once a day, to improve patient compliance and drug efficacy, and to reduce cost.
- When selecting the drug(s), doctors should pay special attention to the patient's race, other diseases and therapies, ability to pay for the drugs, and desired quality of life. The physician will also consider the drug's efficacy and side effects, and its ability to prevent damage to organs such as the heart, brain, or kidney.

One Medicine, Three Names

You've undoubtedly noticed that the drugs your doctor prescribes have two names. One is technical-sounding and often difficult to pronounce (like amlodipine), while the other is more pronounceable, and maybe even flashy (such as Norvasc).

Actually, all drugs have three names. First there is the chemical name, something like 1-[(2S)-3-mercapto-2-methylpropionyl]-L-proline. The chemical name is the first name a drug receives as it's being developed.

Next is the generic or "official" name. Hydrochlorothiazide, propranolol, and lisinopril are the generic names of three antihypertensive medications.

Finally, there's the trade name, the much more easy-to-pronounce name most nondoctors use when talking about their medicines. In fact, some of the trade names sound like they were developed with an eye toward marketing: Dyna Circ sounds like it's going to give you dynamic circulation, Procardia suggests that it will work hard for your heart, and Accupril sound likes it's going to be very accurate. The trade name is also referred to as the brand name.

Some drugs have more than one brand name; that is, the generic drug is offered by more than one pharmaceutical company. For example, hydrochlorothiazide can be purchased as Oretic, Esidrix, and HydroDIURIL.

Here's a little trick that will help you tell if a drug name is the generic name or the trade name: Generic names begin with a lower case letter, while trade names are capitalized and often followed by ®, which signifies that the name is a registered trademark (e.g., amlodipine is the generic name; Norvasc® is the trade name).

THE ANTIHYPERTENSIVE DRUGS: PROS AND CONS

Let's take a brief look at each of the classes of antihypertensive drugs, their benefits and drawbacks.

As you read through the discussion and charts below, you'll see medical terms you may not be familiar with. These words are defined at the end of this chapter.

DIURETICS

Sometimes known as water pills, these drugs are designed to help the body get rid of excess fluid via the urine. They do so by inhibiting the reabsorption of sodium in the areas of the kidneys known as tubules. This slightly reduces the amount of fluid in the blood and extracellular areas, which, in turn, may reduce the cardiac output, or the amount of blood the heart pumps with each beat. Over the long run, the major antihypertensive effect of diuretics is to reduce the systemic vascular resistance, which reduces blood pressure.

Diuretics are used alone in patients with mild to moderate hypertension, or in combination with other types of drugs in more severe cases. There are many different diuretics available today, including:

• Thiazide diuretics, such as hydrochlorothiazide and chlorthalidone, which are mild diuretics that reduce the blood pressure, systemic vascular resistance, and blood volume.

• Loop diuretics, such as Lasix, Bumex, and Demadex, which get their name from the fact that they work primarily in a portion of the kidneys called the loop of Henle.

• Potassium-sparing diuretics, such as triamterene and spironolactone, which don't cause the body to lose as much potassium as the other diuretics do.

- Combination diuretics, which combine the beneficial properties of different types of diuretics.

The major differences between the various diuretics have to do with the area in the kidney they target, how long they last, how powerfully they act, and, of course, their potential side effects.

When treating essential hypertension, the best approach is to start with lower doses of diuretics,[4] then adjust them as necessary. Generally speaking, diuretics are fairly well tolerated. However, patients with anuria (inability to urinate, low or no urinary output) or with a known allergy to the drugs should not take diuretics.

In general, diuretics are relatively inexpensive. They work best in volume-dependent (low-renin) hypertension, normal-renin hypertension, in African-Americans, and the elderly.

Diuretics

Generic Name (*Trade Name or Names*)	Type of Diuretic	Typical Daily Starting Dose	Potential Adverse Effects Include	You Should Not Take This Drug If You Have ...
hydrochlorothiazide (*Oretic, Esidrix, HydroDIURIL*)	thiazide	6.25–25 mg	Excessive calcium, glucose, lipids and uric acid in the blood; inadequate potassium, magnesium, and sodium in the blood; metabolic alkalosis; insufficient fluid in the blood and low blood pressure upon standing up	Inability to urinate, or little or no urinary output; hypersensitivity to sulfonamide derivatives

If Medicine Is Necessary

chlorothiazide (*Diuril*)	thiazide	250 mg	See hydrochlorothiazide	See hydrochlorothiazide
cyclothiazide (*Anhydron*)	thiazide	1–2 mg on alternate days	See hydrochlorothiazide	See hydrochlorothiazide
Methyclothiazide (*Euduron*)	thiazide	2.5–5 mg	See hydrochlorothiazide	Renal decompensation, hypersensitivity
Polythiazide (*Renese*)	thiazide	1–4 mg	See hydrochlorothiazide	See hydrochlorothiazide
chlorthalidone (*Hygroton, Thalitone*)	thiazide	12.5–25 mg	Inadequate magnesium in the blood; hyperlipidemia	See hydrochlorothiazide
bumetadine (*Bumex*)	loop	1–2 mg	Excessive uric acid in the blood; inadequate potassium in the blood; ototoxicity, muscle pain, muscle tenderness, dizziness, low blood pressure, weakness	See hydrochlorothiazide
ethacrynic acid (*Edecrin*)	loop	50–100 mg	Excessive uric acid in the blood; gastrointestinal problems may occur with large doses	Inability to urinate, or little or no urinary output

Generic Name (Trade Name or Names)	Type of Diuretic	Typical Daily Starting Dose	Potential Adverse Effects Include	You Should Not Take This Drug If You Have ...
torsemide (*Demadex*)	loop	5 mg	Excessive uric acid and sugar in the blood; inadequate potassium in the blood; dizziness, headache, nausea, weakness, vomiting, excessive urination, and thirst	Inability to urinate, or little or no urinary output; hypersensitivity
furosemide (*Lasix*)	loop	20–40 mg	Inadequate magnesium and potassium in the blood; fluid and electrolyte imbalance, diarrhea, lowered HDL ("good") cholesterol	Inability to urinate, or little or no urinary output; excessive nitrogen compounds in the blood
triamterene (*Dyrenium*)	potassium-sparing	100 mg twice a day	Excessive sugar and potassium in the blood; abnormalities of red or white blood cells, or platelets; increased skin sensitivity to sunlight, skin rash, metabolic acidosis	
spironolactone (*Aldactone*)	potassium-sparing	50–100 mg	Excessive potassium in the blood; inadequate sodium in the blood; breast development in men; menstrual irregularity, amenorrhea, postmenopausal bleeding, gastrointestinal problems, impotence, fever, rash	Excessive potassium in the blood; inability to urinate, or little or no urinary output; poorly functioning kidneys

amiloride (*Midamor*)	potassium-sparing	5–10 mg	See triamterene	Excessive potassium in the blood; should not be used in combination with other potassium-sparing medicines in people with impaired kidney function
metolazone (*Zaroxolyn, Diulo*)	quinazoline derivative	2.5–5 mg	Excessive sugar, uric acid, calcium and nitrogen compounds in the blood; inadequate amount of sodium, potassium, and magnesium in the blood	Renal insufficiency
indapamide (*Lozol*)	indoline derivative	1.25–2.5 mg	Excessive uric acid in the blood; inadequate amount of potassium, magnesium, and sodium in the blood	

CENTRAL ALPHA AGONISTS

These drugs are designed to stimulate a part of the brain stem called the central postsynaptic $alpha_2$ receptor. Doing so reduces the amount of sympathetic nervous system activity that would otherwise tend to increase blood pressure. The net result is a drop in the systemic vascular resistance, which lowers blood pressure.

There are four central alpha agonists in use today:

- clonidine, sold under the trade name *Catapres*
- guanabenz, sold under the trade name *Wytensin*

- guanfacine, sold under the trade name *Tenex*
- methyldopa, sold under the trade name *Aldomet*

Overall, the central alpha agonists work well, and the members of the group are all about equally effective, but their use is limited due to side effects when given in higher doses. Some people taking clonidine, guanabenz, or guanfacine may excrete more sodium in their urine (natriuresis). When your physician chooses one over the other, he or she will probably be thinking about how long a given drug lasts, how much it costs, and which side effects it triggers. Central alpha agonists can be effective when used alone, as well as when combined with other types of antihypertensives.

Central Alpha Agonists

Generic Name (*Trade Name or Names*)	Typical Daily Starting Dose	Potential Adverse Effects Include	You Should Not Take This Drug If You Have . . .
clonidine (*Catapres*) TTS patch for skin	0.1 mg TTS #1 TTS #2 TTS #3 once per week	Sedation, drowsiness, dry mouth, dizziness, weakness, headache, irregular heartbeat, constipation	Sick sinus syndrome, AV block (2nd or 3rd degree)
guanabenz (*Wytensin*)	16 mg	Dry mouth, sedation, drowsiness, fatigue, impotence, rebound and overshot hypertension, dizziness, weakness, headache, constipation	Pregnancy

guanfacine (*Tenex*)	1 mg	Sedation, drowsiness, dry mouth, dizziness, weakness, headache, irregular heartbeat, constipation	See clonidine
methyldopa (*Aldomet*)	250–500 mg twice a day	Fatigue, drowsiness, sedation, dry mouth, impotence, hepatitis, depression	Active liver disease

BETA BLOCKERS

Beta blockers slow the heart rate, which reduces the cardiac output, but may increase the systemic vascular resistance. They also interfere with the body's ability to increase blood pressure through the renin-angiotensin-aldosterone system. How well the beta blockers work depends on who's taking them. That is, they are most effective in patients with high-renin and normal-renin hypertension, and not nearly as effective in the elderly or in African-Americans.

Beta Blocker Side Effects

When compared to each other, the various beta blockers appear to lower hypertension equally well, but produce more side effects than other classes of drugs. These potential side effects may be significant:

Heart

- Congestive heart failure
- Reduced cardiac output
- Dyspnea (difficulty breathing or shortness of breath)

- Bradycardia (slow heart rate)
- Heart block

Central Nervous System

- Fatigue
- Lethargy
- Weakened memory
- Drowsiness
- Mental depression
- Disorientation
- Insomnia
- Headaches
- Dizziness
- Paresthesia

Gastrointestinal

- Nausea
- Diarrhea
- Constipation
- Flatulence
- Colitis

Respiratory

- Wheezing
- Worsening of asthma and chronic obstructive pulmonary disease
- Bronchospasm

Peripheral Vascular Constriction

- Raynaud's phenomenon (discoloration, burning, tingling, pain and/or numbness in the fingers, toes or nose triggered by stress or cold temperatures)
- Claudication (limping or lameness)
- Cold extremities

Other

- Hyperglycemia
- Reduction of HDL ("good") cholesterol
- Elevation of LDL ("bad") cholesterol
- Elevation of blood fats (triglycerides)
- Postural hypotension (abnormally low blood pressure leading to lightheadedness when you stand up)
- Impotence, decreased libido
- Muscle fatigue
- Inadequate amount of potassium in the bloodstream (hyperkalemia)

Reasons Not to Take Beta Blockers

If you have any of the following conditions, you should avoid beta blockers:

- Sinus bradycardia (slow heart rate)
- Greater than first degree heart block
- Cardiogenic shock (low cardiac output associated with a heart attack)
- Bronchial asthma
- Chronic obstructive pulmonary disease
- Hypersensitivity to the medicine

Beta Blockers

Generic Name (*Trade Name or Names*)	Typical Daily Starting Dose
acebutolol (*Sectral*)	400 mg
atenolol (*Tenormin*)	25–50 mg
betaxolol (*Kerlone*)	10 mg
metoprolol (*Lopressor*)	50 mg once or twice daily
metoprolol (*Toprol XL*)	50–100 mg
nadolol (*Corgard*)	40 mg
carteolol (*Cartrol*)	2.5 mg
penbutolol (*Levatol*)	10 mg
pindolol (*Visken*)	10 mg twice a day
propranolol (*Inderal, Inderal LA*)	40 mg
timolol (*Blocadren*)	10 mg

DIRECT VASODILATORS

These drugs directly relax the arteries, lowering the systemic vascular resistance. However, if they're used alone, without other types of antihypertensive medications, there will be reflex increases in the heart rate, and fluid retention with swelling (edema).

Direct Vasodilators

Generic Name (*Trade Name or Names*)	Typical Daily Starting Dose	Potential Adverse Effects Include	You Should Not Take This Drug If You Have . . .
hydralazine (*Apresoline*)	10 mg four times a day	Abnormally low blood pressure upon standing up, headaches, reflex tachycardia, nausea, palpitations, fatigue, fluid retention, nasal congestion, systemic lupus erythematosus	Aortic aneurysm, coronary artery disease, mitral valve or rheumatic heart disease
minoxidil (*Loniten*)	5 mg	Increased hair growth on the body, fluid retention, weight gain, precipitation of angina, changes on the electrocardiogram, reflex tachycardia	Coronary heart failure, a type of vascular tumor called pheochromocytoma

ALPHA$_1$ BLOCKERS

The walls of your blood vessels are lined with very sensitive nerve cells, called alpha receptors, that receive both chemical and nerve messages prompting vasoconstriction. The alpha$_1$ blockers block these receptors, reducing blood vessel resistance and causing blood pressure to fall.

The combination of an alpha$_1$ blocker plus a modest restriction of sodium intake works well in at least half of the patients with mild hypertension. These drugs reduce levels of cholesterol or blood fats. Side effects are minimal or minor at low doses. They should be used in combination with other antihypertensives, and not as monotherapy (on their own).

Alpha₁ Blockers

Generic Name (*Trade Name or Names*)	Typical Daily Starting Dose	Potential Adverse Effects Include	You Should Not Take This Drug If You Have . . .
doxazosin (*Cardura*)	2–4 mg	Dizziness, increased sweating, fatigue, heart palpitations, sweating	Hypersensitivity to quinazolines
prazosin (*Minipress*)	2–4 mg	Heart palpitations, dizziness, weakness, headaches, abnormally low blood pressure upon standing up	No contraindications
terazosin (*Hytrin*)	2–4 mg	Fainting, abnormally low blood pressure upon standing up, headache, rapid heart rate, swelling, dry mouth, nasal congestion, dizziness, loss of strength or energy	No contraindications

ALPHA-BETA BLOCKERS

These drugs combine the alpha- and beta-blocking effects, reducing the systemic vascular resistance (but making minimal changes in cardiac output). They have a better lipid profile than the pure beta blockers, which means they have less of a negative effect on cholesterol and blood fat. They also produce fewer side effects than the beta blockers.

Alpha-Beta Blockers

Generic Name (*Trade Name or Names*)	Typical Daily Starting Dose	Potential Adverse Effects Include	You Should Not Take This Drug If You Have...
labetalol (*Trandate, Normodyne*)	100 mg twice a day	Coronary heart failure, slow heat rate, fatigue, poor memory, disorientation, nausea, constipation, wheezing	Slow heart rate, heart block (more than 1st degree), cardiogenic shock, certain lung diseases, sensitivity to this drug
carvedilol (*Coreg*)	6.25 mg twice a day	Dizziness, fatigue	NYHA Class IV asthma, AV block (2nd or 3rd degree), a slow heart rate, cardiogenic shock, liver disease
bisoprolol (*Zebeta*)	5 mg	Coronary heart failure, slow heart rate, fatigue, poor memory, disorientation, nausea, constipation, wheezing	Slow heart rate, heart block (more than 1st degree), cardiogenic shock, certain lung diseases, sensitivity to this drug

ANGIOTENSIN-CONVERTING ENZYME INHIBITORS (ACEIs)

Also known as ACE inhibitors, or ACEIs, these drugs interfere with the renin-angiotensin-aldosterone system that raises blood pressure.

As you remember from Chapter 2, the kidneys produce renin, which converts angiotensinogen into angiotensin-I. Angiotensin-I is then converted to angiotensin-II, a powerful blood vessel constrictor that triggers local damage to the arteries, endothelial dysfunction, vascular growth, blood clots, and oxidative stress, among other things. Angiotensin-II also stimulates the secretion of a substance called aldosterone. Aldosterone holds on to sodium and water in the kidneys that normally would be excreted, and increases the blood pressure. Aldosterone also damages the arteries. Clearly, putting the brakes on the renin-angiotensin-aldosterone system can help keep blood pressure and its associated damage under control. The ACE inhibitors do so by preventing the conversion of angiotensin-I to angiotensin-II.

The ACE inhibitors are effective in all types of hypertension. They reduce proteinuria (excessive amounts of protein in the urine), and preserve kidney function. Most people tolerate the ACE inhibitors fairly well, and side effects are relatively minor and infrequent. Cough occurs in about 15 percent of patients.

ACE inhibitors can be effective when used alone, without the aid of other types of antihypertensive drugs. They're also used in combination with many other types of medications.

ACE Inhibitors (ACEIs)

Generic Name (*Trade Name or Names*)	Typical Daily Starting Dose	Potential Adverse Effects Include	You Should Not Take This Drug If You Have . . .
lisinopril (*Prinivil, Zestril*)	5–10 mg	Dizziness, headache, fatigue, diarrhea, cough	Hypersensitivity to the drug, kidney impairment, connective tissue disease, renal artery stenosis
benazepril (*Lotensin*)	10 mg	Headache, dizziness, fatigue, cough, nausea	Similar to lisinopril

captopril (*Capoten*)	25 mg twice a day	Excessive protein in the urine, disturbance in sense of taste, cutaneous rash, leukopenia, renal insufficiency, cough	Renal impairment, renal artery stenosis, connective tissue disease
enalapril (*Vasotec*)	5–10 mg	Similar to captopril	Similar to captopril
fosinopril (*Monopril*)	10–20 mg	Headache, dizziness, fatigue, cough, nausea, diarrhea	Similar to lisinopril
quinapril (*Accupril*)	10–20 mg	Headache, fatigue, nausea, dizziness, cough	Hypersensitivity to the drug
ramipril (*Altace*)	2.5 mg	Headache, dizziness, fatigue, cough, nausea	Hypersensitivity to the drug
moexipril (*Univasc*)	7.5 mg	Headache, dizziness, fatigue, cough, nausea	Hypersensitivity to the drug
trandolapril (*Mavik*)	2 mg	Cough, dizziness, diarrhea, headache, fatigue	Hypersensitivity to the drug
perindopril (*Aceon*)	4 mg	Dizziness, cough, fatigue, headache	Similar to lisinopril

CALCIUM CHANNEL BLOCKERS (CCBS)

Calcium channel blockers slow the movement of calcium into the smooth muscle surrounding the small arteries, making these muscles less able to contract and cause arterial constriction. Calcium channel blockers can be used effectively for mild, moderate, and severe hypertension. The higher the blood pressure is to begin with, the greater the possible therapeutic value of these drugs.

Most people with hypertension respond well to calcium channel blockers, although the best responders are those with low-renin hypertension, African-Americans, and the elderly. Calcium channel blockers work well either as stand-alone drugs or when combined with other kinds of antihypertensive medications.

In general, the calcium channel blockers have a neutral or even favorable effect on lipids (such as blood fats and cholesterol), and are generally well tolerated by patients. They slow the development of atherosclerosis, preserve kidney function, and reduce left ventricular hypertrophy.

Calcium Channel Blockers (CCBs)

Generic Name (*Trade Name or Names*)	Typical Daily Starting Dose	Potential Adverse Effects Include	You Should Not Take This Drug If You Have . . .
amlodipine (*Norvasc*)	5 mg	Dizziness, palpitations, flushing, swelling	Hypersensitivity to the drug
diltiazem SR (*Cardizem SR, Cardizem CD*)	240–360 mg	Headache, heart problems, dizziness, swelling in the ankles and feet	Sick sinus syndrome, AV block (2nd or 3rd degree), severe congestive heart failure, digitalis toxicity, heart attack, pulmonary congestion
diltiazem SR (*Tiazac*)	120–240 mg	A slow heart rate, EKG changes, lack of energy or strength, constipation,	Sick sinus syndrome, AV block (2nd or 3rd degree), severe

		gastric discomfort following eating, palpitations	congestive heart failure, digitalis toxicity, heart attack, pulmonary congestion
diltiazem SR (*Dilacor-XR*)	180–360 mg	Lack of energy or strength, constipation, gastric discomfort following eating, palpitations	Sick sinus syndrome, AV block (2nd or 3rd degree), severe congestive heart failure, digitalis toxicity, heart attack, pulmonary congestion
diltiazem SR (*Tiamate*)	180–360 mg	Lack of energy or strength, constipation, gastric discomfort following eating, palpitations	Sick sinus syndrome, AV block (2nd or 3rd degree), severe congestive heart failure, digitalis toxicity, heart attack, pulmonary congestion
isradipine (*DynaCirc, DynaCirc SR*)	2.5 mg twice a day	Headache, dizziness, swelling, palpitations, fatigue, flushing	Hypersensitivity to the drug
nicardipine (*Cardene, Cardene SR*)	20 mg three times a day	Flushing, headache, pedal edema, lack of energy or strength, palpitations, dizziness, rapid heart rate	Advanced aortic stenosis, hypersensitivity to the drug
nifedipine (*Adalat CC, Procardia XL*)	30 mg	Headache, dizziness, light-headedness, tremor, nervousness, palpitations, leg cramps, fatigue, weakness, nausea, diarrhea, swelling, flushing, abnormally low blood pressure upon standing up, ringing in the ear	Hypersensitivity to the drug

Generic Name (*Trade Name or Names*)	Typical Daily Starting Dose	Potential Adverse Effects Include	You Should Not Take This Drug If You Have . . .
nisoldipine (*Sular*)	20 mg	Similar to nifedipine	Allergy
verapamil (*Calan SR, Isoptin SR, Verelan, Covera-HS*)	240 mg	Constipation, headache, dizziness, light-headedness, weakness, nervousness, itching, flushing, gastric disturbances, hepatitis, abnormally low blood pressure upon standing up, AV block	Sick sinus syndrome, AV block (2nd or 3rd degree), digitalis toxicity, cardiogenic shock
felodipine (*Plendil*)	5 mg	Swelling, headache, flushing, dizziness, lack of energy or strength, irregular heartbeat, fatigue, nausea	Hypersensitivity to the drug

ANGIOTENSIN II RECEPTOR BLOCKERS (ARBs)

Know as ARBs for short, these are the newest class of antihypertensive medications. Just like the ACE inhibitors, the ARBs reduce blood pressure by interfering with the renin-angiotensin-aldosterone system. But whereas the ACE inhibitors block the conversion of angiotensin-I to angiotensin-II, the ARBs prevent angiotensin-II from binding to one of its receptor sites (AT_1R). And if angiotensin-II can't bind to its receptors, it can't pass on the message to constrict the blood vessels. Neither can it stimulate the secretion of aldosterone, which would otherwise trigger the retention of water and sodium in the kidneys, thus pumping up the blood volume.

In general, ARBs are better tolerated than the ACE inhibitors, but equally effective in controlling blood pressure, protecting the kidneys, and reducing proteinuria (protein in the urine).

If Medicine Is Necessary

Angiotensin II Receptor Blockers (ARBs)

Generic Name (*Trade Name or Names*)	Typical Daily Starting Dose	Potential Adverse Effects Include	You Should Not Take This Drug If You Have . . .
candesartan (*Atacand*)	16 mg	Headache, dizziness, upper respiratory infections, inflammation or infection of the pharynx, inflammation of the mucous membranes of the nose	Pregnancy, hypersensitivity to the drug
eprosartan (*Teveten*)	400–800 mg	Similar to other ARBs	Pregnancy, hypersensitivity to the drug
irbesartan (*Avapro*)	150 mg	Diarrhea, gastric discomfort following eating, musculoskeletal trauma, fatigue, upper respiratory infections	Pregnancy, hypersensitivity to the drug
losartan (*Cozaar*)	25–50 mg	Dizziness, lack of energy or strength, headache, cough	Pregnancy, hypersensitivity to the drug
telmisartan (*Micardis*)	40 mg	Upper respiratory infections, back pain, sinusitis, diarrhea, inflammation or infection of the pharynx	Pregnancy, hypersensitivity to the drug
valsartan (*Diovan*)	80 mg	Headache, dizziness, viral infections, fatigue, abdominal pain	Pregnancy, hypersensitivity to the drug
olemarsartan (*Benicar*)	10 mg	Headache, dizziness, viral infections, fatigue, abdominal pain	Pregnancy, hypersensitivity to the drug

POSTGANGLIONIC NEURON INHIBITORS

These drugs are usually poorly tolerated, and are not used to treat hypertension anymore.

Postganglionic Neuron Inhibitors

Generic Name (*Trade Name* or *Names*)	Typical Daily Starting Dose	Potential Adverse Effects Include	You Should Not Take This Drug If You Have . . .
guanadrel (*Hylorel*)	5–50 mg in divided doses	Syncope and volume retention	Congestive heart failure, angina, cerebrovascular disease
guanethidine (*Ismelin*)	10–25 mg	Syncope, volume retention, diarrhea, impotence	A type of vascular tumor called pheochromocytoma, or are simultaneously using epinephrine
reserpine	0.1–0.25 mg	Volume retention	Current or past episodes of depression, active peptic ulcer disease, low blood pressure

SPECIAL NOTE ON MEDICATIONS

In the authors' opinion, diuretics and beta blockers are not the preferred initial therapy for hypertension. ACE inhibitors, angiotensin receptor blockers, and calcium channel blockers are the preferred initial therapy.

QUESTIONS TO ASK YOUR PHYSICIAN BEFORE TAKING *ANY* MEDICINE

Prescribing medicine is—or should be—a collaborative effort. That is, you should not simply put your hand out to receive that little slip of paper from your doctor. Before taking *any* medicine, you should ask a host of questions, including:

- Why this medicine? Why is this drug the right one for me?
- Is this the only medicine that's right for me, or are there other choices?
- Exactly what does the pill, capsule, or caplet look like?
- Exactly how should I take it? How often? At what time? With meals, before eating, after eating, with fluids? Is it okay to take it before driving, sleeping, and so forth?
- Are there any other medicines I should avoid while I'm taking this one?
- Are there any foods I should avoid while I'm taking this drug?
- Are there any vitamins, herbs, or other supplements I should avoid while I'm taking this drug?
- Are there any activities I should avoid while I'm taking this drug? Can I drive, work, have sex, and so on?
- Is there anything about my job or hobbies that will interfere with the effectiveness of this drug or make it dangerous for me?

Make sure your doctor is thoroughly informed about you, your medical history, your lifestyle, and the medications you're taking before he or she prescribes anything for you. Here's a partial list of things to remember to tell him or her about:

- Any allergies
- All medications you're currently taking (including hormones and recreational drugs)

- Any bad reactions you've experienced to *any* medications
- All vitamins, minerals, herbs, or other supplements you're taking or plan to take
- Any over-the-counter medicines, ointments, creams, or weight loss products you're using
- Chemicals, substances, or fumes you come in contact with at work or home
- If you are or intend to become pregnant
- If you are currently breastfeeding
- Your diet, exercise regimen, hobbies, and activities
- Every disease you've ever had, as well as the diseases that have struck your grandparents, parents, and siblings

When prescribing medicine, your doctor needs to know as much as possible about you. The more informed he or she is, the more likely the chance that you'll find the right medication for your unique condition.

DECIPHERING DOCTOR TALK

Here are definitions of some of the "doctor talk" that may be bandied about by your doctor or pharmacist, or that you'll see when you read the package inserts that come with your medications.

- **Aldosteronism**—excessive amounts of the steroid hormone aldosterone in the body. This may lead to retention of sodium, excretion of potassium, elevated blood pressure, kidney disease, and heart problems.
- **Amenorrhea**—lack of menstruation.
- **Angioedema** (also known as angioneurotic edema)—brief swelling of the hands, feet, face, neck, lips, larynx,

genitalia, or viscera, possibly due to infection, emotional stress, or drug or food allergy.
- **Anuria**—inability to urinate, low or no urinary output.
- **Asthenia**—loss of energy and strength.
- **Asystole**—no heartbeat.
- **AV block**—atrioventricular block, or the slowing or stoppage of the electrical impulse that stimulates the heart to beat. Second degree AV block is a partial blockage; 3rd degree AV block is a complete blockage.
- **Azotemia**—too many nitrogen compounds in the blood, a toxic condition caused by inability of the kidneys to do their job.
- **Blood dyscrasias**—abnormalities of the red blood cells, white blood cells, or platelets.
- **Bradycardia**—slow heart rate.
- **Cardiogenic shock**—lowered cardiac output associated with a heart attack and heart failure.
- **Dyspepsia**—gastric discomfort, perhaps bloating, nausea, or heartburn, after eating.
- **Gynecomastia**—abnormal breast development in men.
- **High-renin hypertension**—hypertension with lower blood volume and increased renin.
- **Hypercalcemia**—excessive amounts of calcium in the blood. This may lead to mental confusion, weakness, muscle and abdominal pain.
- **Hyperglycemia**—excessive amounts of sugar (glucose) in the blood. This may lead to diabetes, damage to the blood vessels, and other problems.
- **Hyperkalemia**—excessive amounts of potassium in the blood. This may lead to nausea, muscle weakness, diarrhea, heart changes seen on EKG.

- **Hyperlipidemia**—elevated blood fats (triglycerides), total cholesterol, and LDL ("bad") cholesterol. This may lead to atherosclerosis, heart disease, heart attack, stroke.
- **Hyperreninemia**—excess amounts of the hormone renin in the blood. This may lead to sodium and water retention and blood pressure elevation.
- **Hypersensitivity**—an unusually strong reaction to a foreign substance, similar to allergy.
- **Hypertrichosis**—increased hair growth on the body (but not the scalp).
- **Hyperuricemia**—excessive amounts of uric acid in the blood. This may lead to gout.
- **Hypochloremia**—low levels of chloride in the blood, which can lead to fatigue, heart palpitations, and acid/base problems.
- **Hypochloremic alkalosis**—elevated blood pH (alkaline). This can lead to palpitations, fatigue, and irregular heartbeats.
- **Hypokalemia**—inadequate amounts of potassium in the bloodstream. This may lead to weakness, abnormal heartbeat, and other problems.
- **Hypomagnesemia**—inadequate amounts of magnesium in the bloodstream. This may lead to lethargy, muscle weakness, nausea, and other problems.
- **Hyponatremia**—inadequate sodium concentration in the blood. This may lead to confusion, lethargy, and other problems seen with water intoxication.
- **Impotence**—inability of a man to achieve or maintain an erection. This affects 20 to 25 percent of male patients.
- **Low-renin hypertension**—hypertension with higher blood volume and low renin levels.

- **Metabolic acidosis**—either too little acid or too much base bicarbonate in the body. This can lead to coma and death.
- **Metabolic alkalosis**—either too much acid or too little base bicarbonate in the body. This may lead to severe diarrhea, kidney failure, or other problems.
- **Normal-renin hypertension**—hypertension with normal renin levels.
- **Ototoxicity**—difficulties with hearing and balance.
- **Pancreatitis**—a potentially serious condition in which one or more constituents of the blood are abnormal or are found in abnormal amounts.
- **Paresthesia**—numbness and tingling in the extremities.
- **Pedal edema**—swelling of the ankles and feet.
- **Postural hypotension** (also known as orthostatic hypotension or volume depletion)—low blood pressure when arising from a sitting or lying-down position due to a drop in the amount of fluid in your blood. It causes temporary light-headedness and dizziness.
- **Proteinuria**—excessive amounts of protein, usually albumin, in the urine. An indication of kidney disease.
- **Pruritus**—itching.
- **Pulmonary congestion**—fluid in the lungs.
- **Pulmonary edema**—gathering of fluid in the lungs, often caused by congestive heart failure.
- **Renal decompensation**—kidney damage or failure.
- **Renal insufficiency**—kidney failure or insufficiency.
- **Sick sinus syndrome**—alternating fast/slow heart rate.
- **Sinus arrest**—the upper electrical part of the heart, called the sinus node, stops firing and the heart stops beating.
- **Skin reactions**—inflammation, rash, redness, welts, purpura, or other signs of skin allergy.

- **Stenosis**—narrowing or constriction of a passageway or opening.
- **Tachycardia**—rapid heart rate, perhaps 100 to 150 contractions per minute.
- **Tinnitus**—ringing or tinkling sound in the ear(s).
- **Vasculitis**—an inflammation of the blood vessels.
- **Volume depletion**—See postural hypotension.

Chapter 10

The Future Is Yours

We've covered a lot of ground in this book, delved into the mysteries of high blood pressure and the vascular system, examined the link between nutrients and hypertension, and looked at the drugs designed to combat the disease. Don't worry about trying to master all of the material; just keep these basic ideas in mind:

- Hypertension has reached epidemic proportions in the United States, but it's a remarkably under-treated problem. Some 36 million Americans are walking time bombs, waiting for the excess pressure to blow. And eventually it will, triggering strokes, heart attacks, heart failure, kidney failure, blindness, and other devastating diseases.
- We have many medicines designed to treat elevated blood pressure, including diuretics, calcium channel blockers, beta blockers, ACE inhibitors, and ARBs. These drugs work, and work well, but they can be expensive and many people may not be able to tolerate their side effects.
- Fortunately, there are other approaches, natural medicines

that can lower blood pressure without side effects. Hundreds and hundreds of studies published in the scientific literature detail how various foods, foodstuffs, and supplements can help lower elevated blood pressure just as effectively as the use of a single antihypertensive drug (monotherapy).

For example, the mineral magnesium can reduce the systolic blood pressure by 2 mm Hg or more; allicin, found in garlic, can lower it by 5 to 8 mm Hg; vitamin C can reduce it by 11 mm Hg; and both coenzyme Q_{10} and seaweed can each reduce the pressure by 14 mm Hg. With these natural "medicines" so readily available, there's no reason why millions of hypertensives shouldn't be able to get their conditions under control.

I've put together a list of supplements that have demonstrated an ability to reduce elevated pressure. Here are the ingredients in what I call the VasoGuard Therapy:

Mixed omega-3s (DHA and EPA)	2 gm
Celery seed powder	500 mg
Potassium (as citrate)	20 mg
Vitamin B_6	100 mg
Natural mixed vitamin E	200 IU
Vitamin C (as calcium ascorbate)	500 mg
Garlic powder	250 mg
Taurine	1,500 mg
Natural lycopene tomato extract	5 mg
Biotin	800 mcg
CoEnzyme Q_{10} (Q-Gel®)	50 mg
Lipoic acid	100 mg
Magnesium (as carbonate/sulfate)	185 mg
Calcium (as sulfate)	75 mg

- The VasoGuard Therapy is enhanced by the modified DASH diet I have designed for my patients at the Hypertension Institute. This is a specially tailored version of the DASH-I and DASH-II diets, the only antihypertensive diets accepted by the Joint National Committee on Prevention, Detection, Evaluation, and Treatment of High Blood Pressure, as well as the World Health Organization, the American Heart Association, the American Society of Hypertension, and other major organizations. The modified DASH includes more protein, vegetables, and "good" fat but slightly fewer grains, fruits, and dairy products than the "regular" DASH diets. I've found that it works well for my patients and is tasty and easy to follow, so I can recommend it with great confidence.
- The modified DASH diet, exercise, weight loss, and the VasoGuard Therapy are the mainstays of my natural approach to treating hypertension. All of these elements are backed by solid science, and I've seen them work wonders in my patients. But they're just part of my overall plan for getting you back on the road to good health.

1. *See your physician.* This first step is a must. See your doctor regularly, have him or her monitor your blood pressure, and discuss the changes you'd like to make in your diet, weight, exercise regimen, and lifestyle. It's better to be safe, so keep checking with your physician, and always let him or her know what you're doing.

2. *Adopt the modified DASH diet.* This safe and sane diet can lower elevated blood pressure safely, naturally and significantly. The DASH alone may be all you need.

3. *Use the VasoGuard Therapy.*

4. *Exercise regularly.* Regular exercise reduces elevated blood pressure. Be sure to check with your physician before beginning or changing your regimen; then start sweating!

5. *Maintain your ideal weight.* Those excess pounds you've been carrying around may be pushing up your pressure. Drop the pounds, and your pressure will fall.

6. *De-stress your life.* Stress puts the heat on your blood pressure and overall health. Learn to release stress and relax.

7. *Reduce your alcohol intake to a reasonable level.* If you have hypertension, it is safest to set alcohol aside permanently. If you do drink, limit yourself to less than 20 grams per day—that's about the amount of alcohol you'll find in 24 ounces of beer, 10 ounces of wine, or 2 ounces of hard liquor. (Red wine is probably the best option.)

8. *Cut back on the caffeine.* Limit yourself to less than 100 mg of caffeine per day, or roughly the amount in a 6-ounce cup of brewed coffee, or slightly more than 2 cups of black tea.

9. *Say goodbye to smoking and tobacco.* No smoking. No tobacco of any kind. Ask your doctor how to stop.

10. *Use standard medicines as necessary.* Although natural approaches can and do work for millions of people, there are some who will still need medications. And there are others who will need to remain on their medicines while they are getting into the program and waiting for its good effects to show. But taking medicine doesn't mean that you're a failure. It means you're a success, for you're doing what you need to do to keep the problem under control.

If you're one of the 36 million Americans with uncontrolled hypertension, you can use what you've learned in this book to stop this disease before it stops you. If you're one of the approximately 14 million using drugs to keep your blood pressure under control, you may be able to use the information to cut back on your medications, or eliminate them entirely. Can it really be done? Yes. I've seen many people take back control of their health and their lives. I truly believe that armed with knowledge and determination, you *can* make a positive difference in your health and in your life.

Appendix

A Closer Look at the Studies

In this all-too-brief appendix, we'll take a closer look at the scientific evidence supporting the antihypertensive effects of selected substances. What you'll be reading comes directly from my article titled "The Role of Vascular Biology, Nutrition and Nutraceuticals in the Prevention and Treatment of Hypertension," which appeared in the April 2002 issue of the *Journal of the American Nutraceutical Association*.[169] This is a highly technical discussion intended for physicians and other health professionals.

Unfortunately, space constraints limit this appendix to a portion of that article. Thus, I'll only be able to present the scientific evidence supporting the efficacy of key ingredients of my VasoGuard Therapy: celery, vitamin B_6, vitamin E, vitamin C, garlic, taurine, lycopene, coenzyme Q_{10}, and alpha lipoic acid. I've omitted the discussions of potassium, magnesium, and calcium, as their value is already accepted by the major medical and health organizations. This will allow me to concentrate on some of the lesser-known and less-accepted substances. These substances are discussed below in alphabetical order, and the references are listed at the end of this appendix.

ALPHA LIPOIC ACID (ALA)

Alpha lipoic acid (ALA) is a potent and unique thiol compound antioxidant that is both water- and lipid-soluble.[10] Alpha lipoic acid helps to recirculate tissue and blood levels of vitamins and antioxidants in both lipid and water compartments such as vitamin C and vitamin E, glutathione, and cysteine.[10,125,126] To date, only animal studies in the SHR have been performed to determine the effects of ALA on the vasculature and BP.[10,125,127] Vasdev et al.[125] administered 500 mg/kg/day in their feed, which was equivalent to 26 mg/kg body weight of ALA to the SHR for 9 weeks. There was a significant decrease in SBP ($p<0.001$), as well as reduction in cytosolic and platelet, calcium, glucose, insulin levels, tissue aldehyde conjugates in the liver, kidney, and aorta. Most important, there was evidence of structural improvement in the vasculature with reduced vascular damage, hypertensive VSMH, and atherosclerotic changes. The reduction in SBP in the ALA-treated SHR was from a mean of 180 mm Hg to 140 mm Hg ($p<0.001$); whereas the untreated SHR had an increase in SBP from a baseline of 180 mm Hg to 195 mm Hg over the 9-week study period. The decrease in BP was gradual and did not show a further decrease after 5 weeks of ALA treatment.

The vascular changes in the kidneys of the untreated SHR showed hyperplasia of the smooth muscle, thickening and narrowing of the lumina of the small arteries and arterioles, vacuoles, and PAS-positive material in the walls of the arteries. On the other hand, the ALA-treated SHR kidneys had minimal smooth muscle cell hyperplasia, minimal thickening of the wall, and no narrowing of the lumina in the small arteries and arterioles. Thus, ALA attenuated the renal vascular hyperplasia in the SHR. In this study of the SHR, ALA reduced blood pressure and biochemical and histologic changes. The dose that would be required for an average 70 kg human patient would be about 2,000 mg per day of ALA. However, it should be emphasized that no dose response study in human hypertension has been done to date.

The mechanisms by which ALA reduces BP and promotes improvement in vascular function and structure are numerous.[125,126,128–138] It is known that endogenous aldehydes bind sulfhydryl groups (-SH) in membrane proteins that alter membrane calcium channels (especially L-type calcium channels), which increase cytosolic-free calcium, increase vascular tone, SVR, and BP.[125] Thiol compounds, such as ALA and N-acetyl cysteine (NAC), bind these endogenous aldehydes, normalize the membrane calcium channels, and decrease cytosolic-free calcium. In addition, ALA increases levels of glutathione and cysteine, which bind aldehydes and increase their excretion, and increase antioxidant vitamin levels of ascorbic acid and vitamin E, which improve endothelial dysfunction. ALA acts like a calcium channel blocker (CCB) through these indirect mechanisms.

A Closer Look at the Studies

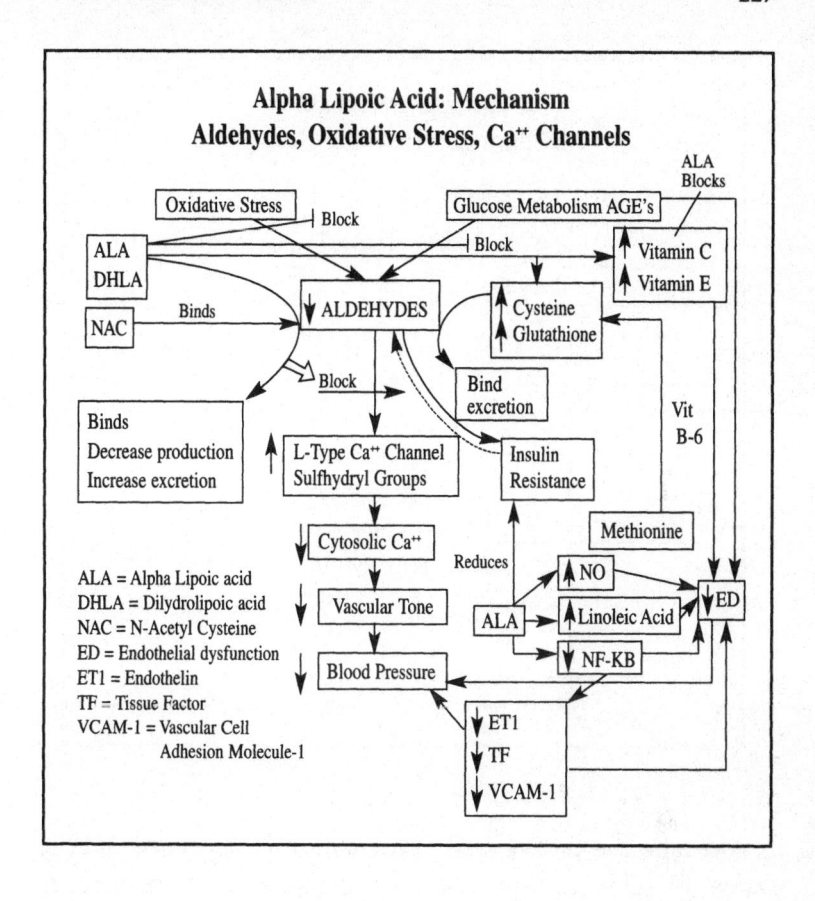

Alpha Lipoic Acid: Mechanism
Aldehydes, Oxidative Stress, Ca^{++} Channels

- Oxidative Stress — Block
- Glucose Metabolism AGE's — Block
- ALA Blocks ↑ Vitamin C, ↑ Vitamin E
- ALA / DHLA
- NAC — Binds
- ↓ ALDEHYDES
- ↑ Cysteine / Glutathione → Bind excretion
- Binds / Decrease production / Increase excretion
- Block → ↑ L-Type Ca^{++} Channel Sulfhydryl Groups
- ↓ Cytosolic Ca^{++}
- ↓ Vascular Tone
- ↓ Blood Pressure
- Insulin Resistance
- Methionine
- ALA Reduces → ↑ NO, ↑ Linoleic Acid, ↓ NF-KB
- Vit B-6
- ↓ ED
- ↓ ET1, ↓ TF, ↓ VCAM-1

ALA = Alpha Lipoic acid
DHLA = Dilydrolipoic acid
NAC = N-Acetyl Cysteine
ED = Endothelial dysfunction
ET1 = Endothelin
TF = Tissue Factor
VCAM-1 = Vascular Cell Adhesion Molecule-1

Alpha Lipoic Acid
Mechanism: Vascular Biology

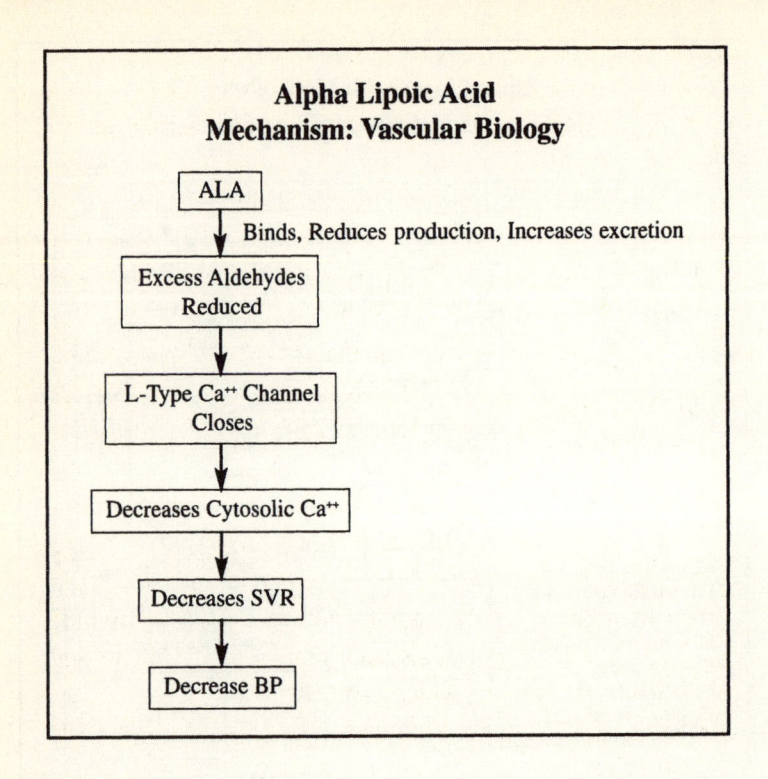

ALA → (Binds, Reduces production, Increases excretion) → Excess Aldehydes Reduced → L-Type Ca^{++} Channel Closes → Decreases Cytosolic Ca^{++} → Decreases SVR → Decrease BP

A detailed summary of the mechanism of action of ALA is shown in Table 1. Glutathione, which supplies 90 percent of nonprotein thiols in the body, is depleted in SHR and human hypertension; thus, ALA, by increasing levels significantly, reducing aldehydes, and closing L-type calcium channels in cell membranes, may reduce vascular tone, SVR, and BP.[131–135]

Table 1

Alpha Lipoic Acid (ALA): Mechanism of Action

1. Increases levels of glutathione, cysteine, vitamins C and E.[125,130]
2. Binds endogenous aldehydes, reduces production, and increases excretion.[125,128,129,130]
3. Normalizes membrane calcium channels by providing sulfhydryl groups (-SH), which reduces cytosolic-free calcium, SVR, vascular tone, and BP. DHLA is redox partner of ALA.[125]
4. Improves insulin sensitivity and glucose metabolism, reduces advanced glycosylation and products (AGEs), and thus aldehydes.[125,128,129,131-135]
5. Increases NO levels, stability, and duration of action via increase in nitrosothiols such as S-nitrosocysteine and S-nitroglutathione which carry NO.[137]
6. Reduces cytokine-induced generation of NO (iNOS).[126,127,137]
7. Inhibits release and translocation of NF-KB from cytoplasm into nucleus of cell, which decreases controlled gene transcription and regulation of endothelin-I, Tissue Factor, VCAM-1.[126,127]
8. Improves ED through beneficial effects on NO, AGEs, vitamins C and E, glutathione, cysteine, endothelin, Tissue Factor, VCAM-1, linoleic and myristic acids.[125,126,128,129,131-135,137,138]
9. Reduces monocyte binding to endothelium (VCAM-1).[126,132]
10. Increases linoleic acid and reduces myristic acid.[130]

CELERY

Animal studies have demonstrated a significant reduction in BP using a component of celery oil, 3-N-butyl phthalide.[164,165] There was a dose response relationship in SBP with a 24 mm Hg fall (14%) ($p<0.05$) in the Sprague-Dawley hypertensive rat model.[165] Significant decreases in plasma norepinephrine, epinephrine, and dopamine were also highly dose-dependent. Celery, celery extract, and celery oil contain apigenin, which relaxes VSM, CCB-like substances and components that inhibit tyrosine hydroxylase, which reduces plasma catecholamine levels, and lowers SVR and BP.[165, 166] Consuming 4 stalks of celery per day, 8 teaspoons of celery juice 3 times daily, or its equivalent in extract form of celery seed (1,000 mg twice a day), or oil (½ to 1 teaspoon 3 times daily in tincture form) seems to provide a similar antihypertensive effect in human essential hypertension.[139,166,167,168] In a Chinese study of 16 hypertensive subjects, 14 had significant reductions in BP.[166,167,168] Celery also has diuretic effects that may reduce BP.[166,167,168] In addition, celery has been used to treat CHF, fluid retention, anxiety, insomnia, gout, and diabetes.[166,167,168]

COENZYME Q$_{10}$ (UBIQUINONE)

Coenzyme Q$_{10}$ (CoQ$_{10}$) is a potent lipid phase antioxidant, free radical scavenger, co-factor, and coenzyme in mitochondrial energy production and oxidative phosphorylation that regenerates vitamins E, C, and A, inhibits oxidation of LDL, membrane phospholipids, DNA, mitochondrial proteins, lipids, reduces TC and TG, raises HDL-C, improves insulin sensitivity, reduces fasting, random and postprandial glucose, lowers SVR, lowers BP, and protects the myocardium from ischemic reperfusion injury.[1,48,67,106–113,170] CoQ_{10} improves mitochondrial energy production, enhancing myocardial infusion with improved diastolic function, left ventricle (LV) function, left ventricle wall tension (LVWT), and NYHA (New York Heart Association) class for CHF.[48,170]

Serum levels of CoQ_{10} decrease with age and are lower in patients with diseases characterized by oxidative stress such as hypertension, CHD, hyperlipidemia, DM, atherosclerosis, and in those who are involved in aerobic training, patients on total parenteral nutrition (TPN), those with hyperthyroidism, and patients who take statin drugs.[48,106,111] Enzymatic assays showed a deficiency of CoQ_{10} in 39% of 59 patients with essential hypertension versus only 6% deficiency in controls ($p<0.01$).[114] There is a high correlation of CoQ_{10} deficiency and hypertension. Most foods contain minimal CoQ_{10}, which is primarily found in meat and seafood. Supplements are needed to maintain normal serum levels in many of these disease states and in some patients taking statin drugs for hyperlipidemia.[48]

Numerous animal studies in SHR, uninephrectomized rats treated with saline or deoxycortisone, and in experimentally induced hypertension in dogs have demonstrated significant reductions in BP following oral administration of CoQ_{10} at doses of 60 mg per day or more.[115–118]

Human studies have also demonstrated significant and consistent reductions in BP in hypertensive subjects following oral administration of 100 mg to 225 mg per day of CoQ_{10}.[71,106,108,109,113,170] Digiesi et al.[106] studied 26 hypertensive subjects with an average BP of 164.5/98.1 mm Hg given CoQ_{10}, 50 mg oral bid for 10 weeks. The SBP fell from 164.5 mm Hg to 146.7 mm Hg, an 11% reduction ($p<0.001$). The DBP was reduced from 98.1 mm Hg to 86.1 mm Hg, a

12% reduction ($p<0.001$). The CoQ_{10} serum levels increased by .97 ug/ml ($p<0.02$), which was highly correlated with the BP reduction. In addition, the twenty-four-hour ABM showed significant reductions in SBP and DBP of 18 mm Hg and 10 mm Hg respectively ($p<0.001$). The TC fell 10 mg% ($p<0.005$), HDL rose 2 mg% ($p<0.01$), and SVR fell 29% ($p<0.02$). There was no significant change in plasma renin activity (PRA), serum K^+, serum Na^+, urinary K^+, or Na^+ or urine aldosterone. Finally, the serum endothelin level, EKG, and echo were not significantly different.

Langsjoen et al.[170] placed 109 hypertensive subjects taking antihypertensive medications on 225 mg per day of CoQ_{10} for four months and demonstrated significant reductions in mean SBP from 159 to 147 mm Hg, a reduction of 12 mm Hg ($p<0.001$), and mean DBP from 94 mm Hg to 85 mm Hg, a reduction of 9 mm Hg ($p<0.001$). Serum CoQ_{10} levels were adjusted to an average of 3.02 ug/ml, but all subjects had levels therapeutic at >2.0 ug/ml. The CoQ_{10} dose varied from 75 to 360 mg per day. There was improvement in diastolic LV function, LVWT, LVH, and NYHA class ($p<0.001$), thought to be mediated secondary to a neurohormonal response with reduction in serum catecholamines and a fall in BP. In addition, improved bioenergetics were noted with improved adrenal function and vascular endothelial function.[119] About 51% of subjects were able to discontinue between one to three antihypertensive drugs (37% stopped one drug, 11% stopped two drugs, 4% stopped three drugs) at an average of 4.4 months after starting CoQ_{10}. No side effects were noted. The reduction in drug use by category was 16.7% decrease in digitalis, 40% decrease in diuretics, 59% decrease in beta blockers, 27.5% decrease in calcium channel blockers, 31.7% decrease in angiotensin-converting enzyme inhibitors, and a 35% decrease in other antihypertensive drugs.[170]

Yamagami et al.[120] observed a CoQ_{10} deficiency in 29 subjects with essential hypertension and found significant improvement in their BP and correction of the CoQ_{10} deficiency following oral intake of 1–2 mg/kg/day. Tsuyusaki et al.[121] found that CoQ_{10} at 30 mg per day when added to a beta blocker reduced the negative inotropic effect and lowered BP. Richardson et al.[122] demonstrated a significant reduction in systolic and diastolic blood pressure in 16 subjects with essential hypertension on 60 mg per day of CoQ_{10} treatment for 12 weeks as well as normalization of their cardiac output. Hamada et al.[123] did not see a significant change in BP in 12 hypertensive subjects treated with CoQ_{10} at 60 mg per day for 4 weeks, but the negative inotropic effect of a beta blocker was reduced, and the malaise and fatigue in the patients improved. Yamagami et al.[119] showed a significant decrease in SBP in 20 essential hypertensive subjects with low CoQ_{10} levels (less than 0.9 ug/ml) who were randomized to receive either placebo or CoQ_{10} at 100 mg per day for 12 weeks. The BP decreased significantly in the CoQ_{10} group between 8 to 12 weeks. Montaldo et al.[124] studied 15 hypertensive subjects on 100 mg per day of CoQ_{10} for 12 weeks and noted a significant reduction in BP at rest and exercise as well as a significant improvement in myocardial stroke work index.

Digiesi et al.[113] in 1992 evaluated 10 subjects with essential hypertension treated with oral CoQ_{10}, 50 mg BID for 10 weeks. The SBP fell from 161.5 +/− 5.1 mm Hg to 142.2 +/− 5.3 mm Hg ($p<0.001$), and the DBP fell from 98.5 +/− 1.7 mm Hg to 83.1 +/− 2.0 mm Hg ($p<0.001$). Plasma CoQ_{10} levels increased from 0.69 +/− 0.1 ug/ml to 1.95 +/− 0.3 ug/ml ($p<0.02$). In addition, TC decreased from 227 +/− 24 mg% to

203.7 +/− 20.6 mg% (p<0.01), and serum HDL cholesterol increased from 42 +/− 3.0 mg% to 45.9 +/− 3.0 mg% (p<0.01). The PRA, urine K⁺, Na⁺, and aldosterone did not change. The SVR decreased significantly and correlated directly with BP reduction.

Digiesi et al. in 1990[109] evaluated 18 subjects with essential hypertension, off all antihypertensive drugs, treated with CoQ_{10}, 100 mg orally per day for 10 weeks versus placebo, then subjects were crossed over to the opposite study group after a 2-week treatment suspension. Compared to the placebo subjects, there was a significant reduction in SBP from 166 +/− 2.6 mm Hg to 156 +/− 2.25 mm Hg, and DBP from 102.9 +/− 1.2 mm Hg to 95.2 +/− 1.04 mm Hg, both significant at p<0.001. The placebo group had no significant reduction in BP. The antihypertensive effect of CoQ_{10} was observed during the third and fourth week of treatment, remained constant for the entire duration of treatment, and ceased 7 to 10 days after the end of drug treatment. No adverse effects were noted.

Recently, Singh et al.[108] evaluated 30 treated hypertensive subjects with CHD treated with CoQ_{10}, 60 mg BID, for 8 weeks versus a vitamin B complex. The CoQ_{10}-treated subjects had a reduction in SBP from 168 +/− 9.6 mm Hg to 152 +/− 8.2 mm Hg (16 mm Hg reduction, p<0.05), and a DBP reduction from 106 +/− 4.6 mm Hg to 97 +/− 4.1 mm Hg (9 mm Hg reduction, p<0.05). In addition, the heart rate fell from 112 +/− 7.8 to 85 +/− 4.8 per minute (p<0.05). Fasting and two-hour insulin fell 45% and 35% respectively (p<0.05), as fasting glucose decreased 33% (p<0.05). Serum TG fell 10 percent and HDL cholesterol increased significantly (p<0.05), lipid peroxides decreased (p<0.05), malondialdehyde fell (p<0.05), and olene conjugates were reduced (p<0.05). Serum vitamins A, C, and E, and beta-carotene levels increased. The only changes in the B-vitamin complex group were increases in vitamin C and beta-carotene ($p<0.05$).

The mechanism of action of CoQ_{10} includes a reduction in SVR, decreased degradation of membrane phospholipids, decreased membrane phospholipase A_2 activity, membrane-stabilizing activity, decreased catecholamine and aldosterone levels, improved insulin sensitivity, decreased OxLDL, antioxidant effects on endothelium and vascular smooth muscle (VSM) with increased NO, decreased VSM hypertrophy, vasodilation, decreased ED, and improved mitochondrial energy production with less vascular ischemia.[108,109,113,170]

In summary, CoQ_{10} has consistent and significant antihypertensive effects in patients with essential hypertension. The major conclusions from in vitro, animal, and human clinical trials indicate the following:

1. Compared to normotensive patients, essential hypertensive patients have a high incidence of CoQ_{10} deficiency documented by serum levels.

2. Doses of 120 to 225 mg per day of CoQ_{10}, depending on the delivery method and concomitant ingestion with a fatty meal, are necessary to achieve a therapeutic level of over 2 ug/ml. This is usually 1–2 mg/kg/day of CoQ_{10}. The best studied and most bioavailable CoQ_{10} supplement is Q-Gel, (Tishcon Corp., Westbury, New York). Use of this special delivery system allows better absorption and lower oral doses.

3. Patients with the lowest CoQ_{10} serum levels may have the best antihypertensive response to supplementation.

4. The average reduction in BP is about 15/10 mm Hg based on reported studies.

5. The antihypertensive effect takes time to reach its peak level, usually at about four weeks, then BP remains stable. The

antihypertensive effect is gone within two weeks after discontinuation of CoQ_{10}.

6. Approximately 50 percent of patients on antihypertensive drugs may be able to stop between one and three agents. Both total dose and frequency of administration may be reduced.

7. Even high doses of CoQ_{10} have no acute or chronic adverse effects.

Other favorable effects on cardiovascular risk factors include improvement in the serum lipid profile and carbohydrate metabolism with reduced glucose and improved insulin sensitivity, reduced oxidative stress, reduced heart rate, improved myocardial LV function and oxygen delivery, and decreased catecholamine levels.

GARLIC

Good clinical trials utilizing the correct type and dose of garlic have shown consistent reductions in BP in hypertensive patients.[1,10–20] Not all garlic preparations are processed similarly and are not comparable in antihypertensive potency.[21,22] In addition, cultivated garlic (*Allium sativum*),[21,22] wild uncultivated garlic or bear garlic (*Allium urisinum*)[21–31] and aged[7] or fresh garlic will have variable effects.[1,11,12] Mohamadi et al.[22] found that wild garlic had the greatest antihypertensive effect in rats, probably mediated through the reduction in A-II levels, increased NO, and decreased ROS by the higher content of allicin and other compounds. There is a consistent dose-dependent reduction in BP with garlic mediated through the RAAS and the NO system.[22] ALLICIN, a synthetic preparation of an active constituent of garlic, lowered BP, insulin, and TG to a similar degree as enalapril in the Sprague-Dawley Rat Study by Elkayam et al.[32]

Approximately 10,000 mcg of allicin per day, the amount contained in four cloves of garlic (4 grams) is required to achieve a significant BP-lowering effect.[1,11,12] In humans the average reduction in SBP is 5–8 mm Hg.[33]

Garlic contains numerous active compounds that may account for its antihypertensive effects, including gammaglutamyl peptides (natural ACEI),[23,30,31] flavonolic compounds (natural ACEI),[23,31] magnesium (vasodilator and natural CCB),[21,23] ajoenes,[7,21,23] phosphorous,[21,23] adenosine,[25-29] allicin,[7,22] and sulfur compounds.[7] The proposed mechanisms of action of garlic in reducing BP are shown in Table 2. Garlic probably is a natural ACEI and CCB that increases BK and NO-inducing vasodilation, reducing SVR and BP and improving vascular aortic compliance.

Approximately 30 hypertensive clinical trials have been completed to date and 23 reported results with placebo control, 4 used nonplacebo controls, and 3 did not report results.[33] These trials studied BP as the primary outcome and 7 excluded concomitant antihypertensive medications. Significant reductions in DBP of 2–7% were noted in 3 trials and reductions in SBP of 3% in 1 trial when compared to placebo. Other trials reported BP reductions in the garlic-treated subjects (within group comparisons). Many studies did not provide numerical data about BP or did not have an a priori hypothesis regarding BP reduction.

Table 2

> **Garlic: Mechanisms of Action**
> - ACEI (gammaglutamyl peptides, flavonolic compounds)[21–24,30,31]
> - Increases NO[14,22]
> - Decreases sensitivity to NE[14,22]
> - Increases adenosine[14,22,25–29]
> - Vasodilation and reduced SVR[7,22]
> - Inhibits AA metabolites (TxA$_2$)[7,22]
> - Reduces aortic stiffness[7]
> - Magnesium (natural CCB vasodilator)[21,23]
> - Decreases ROS[22]

LYCOPENE (CAROTENOID)

Lycopene is a non-provitamin-A carotenoid, potent antioxidant found in tomatoes and tomato products, guava, pink grapefruit, watermelon, apricots, and papaya in high concentrations.[103] Lycopene has recently been shown to produce a significant reduction in BP, serum lipids and oxidative stress markers.[104,105] Paran et al.[105] evaluated 30 subjects with Stage 1 hypertension, ages 40 to 65, taking no antihypertensive or antilipid medications and treated with a tomato lycopene extract for 8 weeks. The SBP was reduced from 144 to 135 mm Hg (9 mm Hg reduction, p<0.01), and DBP fell from 91 to 84 mm Hg (7 mm Hg reduction, p<0.01). A similar study of 35 subjects with Stage 1 hypertension showed similar results on SBP, but not DBP.[104] Serum lipids were significantly improved in both studies without change in serum homocysteine.

TAURINE

Taurine is a sulfonic beta-amino acid that is considered a conditionally essential amino acid, which is not utilized in protein synthesis, but rather is found free or in simple peptides, with its highest concentration in the brain, retina, and myocardium.[140,141] In cardiomyocytes, it represents about 50% of the free amino acids and has a role of an osmoregulator and inotropic factor and has been used to treat hypertension,[142] hypercholesterolemia, arrhythmias, atherosclerosis, CHF, and other cardiovascular conditions.[140,141,143,144]

Animal studies have shown consistent and significant reductions in BP.[145-155] Taurine inhibited the alcohol-induced hypertension in SHR by reducing acetylaldehyde and changing membrane cation handling.[145] In the SHR-high-sodium model, taurine reduced proteinuria and lowered BP 20–25%,[151] and reduced LVH, urinary epinephrine, and dopamine.[146,155] The DOCA-salt rat model had BP reduction due to decreased sympathetic nervous system (SNS) activity centrally[147,149] due to an opiate-mediated vasodepressor response.[150,153] Taurine increases renal kallikrein[154] and has an anti-atherosclerotic effect.[152]

Human studies have noted that essential hypertensive subjects have reduced urinary taurine as well as other sulfur amino acids.[156,157] Taurine lowers BP[142,143,144,157,158,159] and HR,[144] decreases arrhythmias,[144] CHF symptoms[144] and SNS activity,[142,144] increases urinary sodium[158,160] and decreases PRA, aldosterone,[160] plasma norepinephrine,[159] and plasma and urinary epinephrine.[142,161] This diuretic effect is seen in normal subjects as well as hypertensive and cirrhotics with ascites.[158-161] In doses of 6 grams per day for 3 weeks in 22 healthy, normotensive, male volunteers, taurine reduced SNS activity, urinary epinephrine, TC, and LDL, but increased TG, while BP and BMI did not change significantly.[161] Another study of 31 Japanese males with essential hypertension placed on an exercise program for 10 weeks showed a 26% increase in taurine levels and a 287% increase in cysteine levels. The BP reduction of 14.8/6.6 mm Hg was proportional to both taurine level elevations and plasma norepinephrine reduction.[159] Fujita et al.[142] reduced BP 9/4.1 mm Hg ($p<0.05$) in 19 hypertension subjects given 6 grams of taurine for 7 days.

The mechanisms by which taurine exerts its cardiovascular and antihypertensive effects include diuresis[141,160] and urinary sodium loss,[160] vasodilation,[141] increased atrial natriuretic factor (ANF),[141] reduced homocysteine,[140] improved glucose and insulin sensitivity,[156] increased sodium space,[148] reduced SNS activity and opiate-mediated vasodepressor response,[150,153] increased renal kallikrein,[154] reduced PRA and aldosterone,[160] and a glycine-mediated CNS response with decreases in both BP and HR.[171]

Concomitant use of enalapril with taurine provides additive reductions in BP, LVH, arrhythmias,[162,163] and platelet aggregation.[163] The recommended dose of taurine is 2 to 3 grams per day at which no adverse effects are noted, but higher doses may be needed to reduce BP significantly.[142]

VITAMIN B$_6$ (PYRIDOXINE)

Low serum vitamin B$_6$ levels are associated with hypertension in rats[9,85–89] and humans.[85,90–96] Vitamin B$_6$ is a readily metabolized and excreted water-soluble vitamin.[97] Six different B$_6$ vitamins exist, but pyridoxal 5/phosphate (PLP) is the primary and most potent active form that is produced by rapid hepatic oxidation by pyridoxine phosphate oxidase and pyridoxine

A Closer Look at the Studies

kinase in the presence of zinc and magnes... PLP-dependent enzymes exist that are invol... pathways that include carbohydrate metabolism... biosynthesis and degradation, amino acid metab... biosynthesis, and hormone and neurotransmitter bi... ...sis such as steroid hormones, thyroid hormone, gamma amino butyric acid (GABA), histamine, norepinephrine (NE), and serotonin.[96,97] Vitamin B_6's participation in neurotransmitter and hormone biosynthesis, amino acid reactions with kynureninase, cystathionine synthetase, cystathionase, and membrane L-type calcium channels account for much of its antihypertensive effects.[97,98] Vitamin B_6 (PLP) is involved in the transsulfuration pathway of homocysteine metabolism to cysteine.[97]

Animal studies in specific rat strains have demonstrated an increase in BP, NE, and epinephrine plasma levels, an increase in the NE cardiac turnover, reduced CNS brain stem NE, GABA, and serotonin content that completely reverses after vitamin B_6 repletion.[98] Pyridoxine at 10 mg/kg in B_6-deficient rats (B6DHT) reduced BP from 143 mm Hg to 119 mm Hg within 24 hours ($p<0.05$).[98] In these B6DHT rats, PLP enhanced binding of CCBs to the vascular membrane, indicating that PLP corrects membrane abnormalities and is an endogenous modulator of DHP-sensitive (dihydropyridine-sensitive) calcium channels.[87,99] Low calcium levels and low B_6 levels potentiate BP increases in rats, whereas replacement of both will reduce BP.[9] Vitamin B_6 plus tryptophan reduced BP more than monotherapy with each in rats, probably related to effects on brain stem serotonin and kynurenine.[86] There is a structural similarity of the B_6 vitamins to the DHP-CCBs, and CCBs are most effective in B_6-deficient rats.[85]

Supplemental vitamin B_6 in the diets of prehypertensive, obese, Zucker, and sucrose-induced hypertensive rats, and SHR reduces BP by increasing the synthesis of cysteine from methionine.[100,101,102] Cysteine acts directly on aldehydes and neutralizes their effects. Aldehydes bind sulfhydryl groups of membrane proteins and alter calcium channels (L-type), which increase cytosolic-free calcium, cause VSM constriction, and elevate BP.[102] Aldehydes also induce hyperglycemia and promote insulin resistance.[102] Cysteine is also a precursor of glutathione, which neutralizes aldehydes and further improves BP and glucose metabolism.[102] Thus, vitamin B_6 reduces both movement of calcium into cells (cytosolic Ca^{++}) and decreases intracellular sarcoplasmic reticulum release of calcium.

One human study by Aybak et al.[96] proved that high-dose vitamin B_6 significantly lowered BP. This study compared 9 normotensive men and women with 20 hypertensive subjects, all of whom had significantly higher BP, plasma NE, and HR compared to control normotensive subjects. Subjects received 5 mg/kg/day of vitamin B_6 for 4 weeks. The SBP fell from 167 +/− 13 mm Hg to 153 +/− 15 mm Hg, an 8.4% reduction ($p<0.01$), and the DBP fell from 108 +/− 8.2 mm Hg to 98 +/− 8.8 mm Hg, a 9.3% reduction ($p<0.005$). Plasma NE was reduced from 1.80 +/−.21 nmol/l to 1.48 +/− .32 nmol/l (18% reduction, $p<0.005$); plasma epinephrine fell from 330 +/− 64 pmol/l to 276 +/− 67 pmol/l (16% reduction, $p<0.05$). There was no significant change in heart rate.

The proposed mechanisms of hypertension in vitamin B_6–deficient animals and humans include:[97,98]

1. Central nervous system and brain stem depletion of neurotransmitters such as NE, serotonin, and GABA, which leads to an increase in sympathetic outflow.
2. Increased peripheral SNS activity.

3. Increased VSMC calcium uptake and incr[...]lular calcium release.

4. Increased end organ responsiveness to gluco[...] and mineralocorticoids (aldosterone).

5. Increased aldehyde levels.

6. Insulin resistance.

In summary, vitamin B_6 has multiple antihypertensive effects that resemble those of central alpha agonists (e.g., clonidine), calcium channel blockers (e.g., DHP-CCB-like amlodipine), and diuretics. Finally, changes in insulin sensitivity and carbohydrate metabolism may lower BP in selected hypertensive individuals with the metabolic syndrome of insulin resistance. Chronic intake of vitamin B_6 at 200 mg per day is safe and has no adverse effects. Even doses up to 500 mg per day are probably safe.[97]

VITAMIN C

Vitamin C is a potent water-soluble antioxidant that recycles vitamin E, improves endothelial dysfunction, and produces a diuresis.[10,34-38] Numerous epidemiologic, observational, and clinical studies have demonstrated that the dietary intake of vitamin C or plasma ascorbate concentration in humans is inversely correlated to SBP, DBP, and heart rate.[2,3,5,39-56] Studies in the SHR have shown fairly uniform reductions in BP with vitamin C administration.[57] Long-term epidemiologic and observational follow-up studies in humans also show a reduced risk of CVD, CHD, and CVA with increased vitamin C intake.[47,49,58,59] However, controlled intervention trials have been somewhat less consistent or inconclusive as to the relationship of vitamin C administration and BP.[3,42,49-52,60] Numerous reasons exist for these variable results, including lack of a control group, no baseline BP, small study population, short trial duration, variable vitamin C doses, variable demographics and study population, unknown premorbid vitamin C status or premorbid general vitamin or antioxidant status, concomitant or unknown multivitamin intake and unknown nutritional status, existing concomitant diseases, confounding factors such as smoking, alcohol, weight changes, fiber, etc. were not stated or evaluated, plasma ascorbic acid levels were not measured, the P-value and confidence intervals were not reported, variable BP measurement techniques were employed (clinic or office, home, 24-hour ABM), unknown genetic polymorphisms exist or there was publication bias.[3]

Ness et al.[3] published in 1997 a systematic review of MEDLINE-listed peer review journals on hypertension and vitamin C and concluded that if vitamin C has any effect on BP, it is small. However, in the 18 studies that were reviewed worldwide, 10 of 14 showed a significant BP reduction with increased plasma ascorbate levels and 3 of 5 demonstrated a decreased BP with increased dietary vitamin C.[3] In 4 small, randomized clinical trials of 20 to 57 subjects, 1 had significant BP reduction, 1 had no significant BP reduction, and 2 were not interpretable.[3] In 2 uncontrolled trials, there was a significant reduction in BP.[3]

Koh et al.[54] in 1984 evaluated 23 hypertensive women with a BP range of 140–160/90–100 mm Hg over a 3-month period. Administration of 1 gram of vitamin C per day reduced office SBP 7 mm Hg ($0.05<p<0.10$) and reduced DBP 4 mm Hg ($0.05<p<0.10$). Ceriello et al. in 1991[2] gave IV vitamin C to hypertensive patients with DM and reduced BP significantly.

Trout et al. in 1991[46] gave 1 gram of vitamin C orally to 12 hypertensive subjects in a randomized crossover study for 6 weeks. The plasma ascorbate levels increased by 20 umol/liter (p<0.001), SBP fell 5 mm Hg (p<0.05), and DBP fell 1 mm Hg +/− 2 (NS)

Duffy et al.[42] in 1999 evaluated 39 hypertensive subjects (DBP 90 mm Hg to 110 mm Hg) in a placebo-controlled 4-week study. A 2,000 mg loading dose of vitamin C was given initially followed by 500 mg per day. The SBP was reduced 11 mm Hg (p = 0.03), DBP decreased by 6 mm Hg (p = 0.24), and MAP fell 10 mm Hg (p<0.02). The plasma ascorbate increased to 49 umol/liter at 4 weeks (p<0.001), showing an inverse correlation with MAP and plasma ascorbate levels (p<0.03). There was no change in cyclic GMP (CGMP), urinary 6 keto-prostaglandin-Fl $\propto$ =or urinary 8 epi-prostaglandin-F2 $\propto$.

Fotherby et al. (2000)[53] studied 40 mild hypertensive and normotensive subjects in a double-blind, randomized, placebo-controlled, crossover study for 6 months. Men and women ages 60 to 80 years (mean age 72 +/− 4 years) were given 250 mg vitamin C twice daily for 3 months, then crossed over after a 1-week washout period. The plasma ascorbate increased to 35 umol/liter (p<0.001), but clinic BP did not change significantly. However, the 24-hour ABM showed a significant decrease in SBP 2.0 +/− 5.2 mm Hg (p<0.05), but there was no significant change in DBP. However, the higher the BP, the greater the response to vitamin C. Therefore, when the normotensive or borderline hypertensive subjects were excluded, the BP reduction was more pronounced and significant. A significant increase in HDL-C was seen in women (p<0.007), but not in men. The LDL-C did not change in either group. The conclusion from this study was that vitamin C reduced primarily daytime SBP as measured by 24-hour ABM in hypertensive, but not normotensive, subjects. In the hypertensive subjects, SBP was reduced by 3.7 mm Hg +/− 4.2 mm Hg ($p<0.05$), and DBP fell 1.2 mm Hg +/− 3.7 mm Hg (NS).

Block et al. (2001)[61] in an elegant depletion-repletion study of vitamin C demonstrated a significant inverse correlation of plasma ascorbate levels, SBP, and DBP. During this 17-week controlled diet study of 68 normotensive men ages 39 to 59 years with mean DBP of 73.4 mm Hg and mean SBP of 122.2 mm Hg, vitamin C depletion at 9 mg per day for 1 month was followed by vitamin C repletion at 117 mg per day repeated twice. All confounders were eliminated, including smoking, exercise, alcohol, weight change, and other nutritional intake during the study. Plasma ascorbate was inversely related to DBP ($p<0.0001$, correlation −0.48) and to SBP in logistic regression. Persons in the bottom quartile of plasma ascorbate had a DBP 7 mm Hg higher than those in the top quartile. One fourth of the DBP variance was accounted for by plasma ascorbate alone. Of the other plasma nutrients examined, only ascorbate was significantly and inversely correlated with DBP ($p<0.0001$, $r = -0.48$) for the 5-week plasma ascorbate levels. Each increase at week 5 in the plasma ascorbate level was associated with a 2.4 mm Hg lower DBP at week 9.

Hajjar et al.[62] evaluated 31 subjects with stage 1 hypertension in a double-blind, randomized, placebo, 4-week, run-in trial utilizing 3 doses of vitamin C at 500 mg, 1,000 mg, or 2,000 mg per day for 8 months. The mean age was 62 +/− 2 years, 52% male, 90% white with good compliance of 48 +/− 2%. The SBP fell significantly by 4.5 +/− 1.8 mm Hg ($p<0.05$), and DBP fell by 2.8 +/− 1.2 mm Hg ($p<0.05$) at 1 month and persisted during the study. No dose response was demonstrated. The BP decrease was not significant, but was lower in the vitamin C group. There was no difference in BP response between the three groups ($p = 0.48$), and no significant change in serum lipid levels from baseline or between groups although the vitamin C group had an overall trend to improve lipids: TC (p = 0.75), TG (p = 0.87), HDL (p = 0.32), or LDL (p = 0.52).

Ness et al.[40] evaluated subjects ages 45 to 74 in a population-based cross-sectional analysis and found that an increase in plasma ascorbate of 50 umol/liter reduced BP by 3.6/2.6 mm Hg. Bates et al.[39] in a similar cross-sectional analysis on 914 elderly patients over 65 years of age confirmed that an increase in plasma ascorbate of 50 umol/liter reduced SBP by 7 mm Hg. In most of the epidemiologic studies, there is a clear inverse relationship between plasma ascorbate levels and dietary intake, and BP, with a reduction in SBP of 3.6 to 17.8 mm Hg for each 50 umol/liter increase in plasma ascorbate.[3,39,40,44–48]

In the post hoc analysis in the ADMIT study (Arterial Disease Multiple Intervention Trial),[60] a prospective, double-blind, placebo-controlled study of 363 subjects with PAD (peripheral arterial disease) treated with vitamin C 1,000 mg per day, vitamin E 800 IU/day, and beta-carotene 24 mg per day versus placebo, there was no difference in BP in the normotensive or hypertensive subjects (N = 177). Other studies, however, have shown synergy of combination antioxidants and vitamins in reducing BP, increasing NO, PGE,[1 6,8,63] and PGI^2 levels,[5,53,64,65] and reducing TxA_2 levels. The study by Miller et al.[66] in 297 elderly patients showed no difference in BP in the treated group given vitamin C, E, and beta-carotene versus a placebo group. However, 87% of all subjects were permitted to take their own multivitamins.

In Table 3, we see the Mechanisms of Vitamin C on Blood Pressure.

Table 3

Mechanisms of Vitamin C on Blood Pressure

- Reduces ED and improves EDVD and lowers BP and SVR in HBP, HLP, CHD, smokers[4,10,34–38,40,41,43,53,56,67,68]
- Diuresis[10]
- Increases NO and PGI_2[46,53,69,70]
- Decreases adrenal steroid production[53]
- Improves sympathovagal balance[53,173]
- Decreases cystosolic Ca^{++}[45]
- Antioxidant[10,45]
- Recycles vitamin E, glutathione, uric acid[10,45]
- Reduces neuroendocrine peptides[53,69,70]
- Reduces thrombosis[45,53] and decreases TxA_2[70]
- Reduces lipids (↓TC, ↓LDL, ↓TG, ↑HDL)[53,174,175]
- Reduces leukotrienes[45,46]
- Improves aortic collagen, elasticity, and aortic compliance[61,176]
- Increases cGMP and activates VSM K^+ channels[56]

Vitamin C improves ED in hypertensive[10, 36] and hyperlipidemic[35] patients and reduces BP in a dose-related manner with higher pharmacologic doses.[10,34] The improvement of ED in hypertensive patients occurs in conduit arteries, epicardial coronary arteries, and forearm-resistance arteries.[4,35,67,68] Vitamin C restores NO-mediated flow-dependent vasodilation in patients with CHF.[68] Hypertensive patients exhale less NO than healthy patients.[43] Following vitamin C administration, there is an increase in exhaled NO that correlates with BP reduction, especially SBP.[43] Acute oral or intravenous administration of vitamin C reverses ED and causes acute vasodilation in humans with CHD[37] and in smokers.[38] The multitude of proposed mechanisms for vitamin C in hypertension and other cardiovascular diseases are outlined in Table 3. Grossman et al.[56] proposed recently that ascorbic acid modulates the redox state of soluble guanylyl cyclase, activating cGMP-dependent potassium channels that hyperpolarize VSMC-inducing vasodilation.

Table 4

Vitamin C: Conclusions

1. BP is inversely correlated with vitamin C intake and plasma ascorbate levels in humans and animals in epidemiologic, observational, cross-sectional, and controlled prospective clinical trials.
2. A dose response relationship between lower BP and higher plasma ascorbate levels is suggested:
   A) DBP fell about 2.4 mm Hg per plasma ascorbate quartile in a depletion repletion study.
   B) SBP fell 3.6 to 17.8 mm Hg for each 50 μmol/L increase in plasma ascorbate level.
   C) BP may be inversely correlated to tissue levels of ascorbate.
   D) Doses of 100 to 1,000 mg per day are needed.
3. SBP is reduced proportionately more than DBP, but both are decreased. Twenty-four-hour AMB indicates a predominate daytime SBP reduction and lower HR. Office BP shows a reduction in SBP and DBP as well.
4. The greater the initial BP, the greater the BP reduction.

5. BP is reduced in hypertensives, normotensives, hyperlipidemics, diabetics, and in patients with a combination of these diseases.
6. Improves ED in HBP, HLP, PAD, DM, CHD, CHF, smokers, and in conduit arteries, epicardial coronary arteries, and forearm resistance arteries

VITAMIN E

The relationship of vitamin E and BP has been studied in vitro,[69] extensively in animals (SHR),[72–77] but limited studies have been done in humans.[78,79] Alpha tocopherol inhibits thrombin-induced endothelin secretion in vitro at least partially through protein kinase C (PKC) inhibit ion.[80] Reduced PKC levels reduce vascular smooth muscle (VSM) proliferation through inhibition of activated protein-1 (AP-1) and nuclear factor kappa-B (NFKB). This, in turn, improves ED, lowers SVR, and reduces BP.

Newaz et al.[72] gave gamma tocotrienol 15 mg/kg to SHR and found significant reductions in lipid peroxides in plasma and in blood vessel walls, increased superoxide dismatase (SOD) activity, increased total antioxidant status (TAS), and lowered BP ($p<0.001$). In a similar study, Newaz et al.[73] gave 34 mg/kg of alpha tocopherol to SHR and WKY rats. Lipid peroxide levels were decreased in plasma and in vascular walls, plasma SOD activity increased, TAS increased, and BP fell ($p<0.001$). In a follow-up, dose-response study,[74] Newaz administered alpha tocopherol to SHR in doses of 17 mg/kg, 34 mg/kg or 170 mg/kg. Nitric oxide synthase (NOS) increased significantly ($p<0.01$) only at the 34 mg/kg dose, and BP fell the most at the 34 mg/kg dose ($p<0.001$).

Other animal studies have shown beneficial results of alpha tocopherol on hypertension and stroke in the SHR,[75] membrane fluidity and BP in SHR and WKY rats,[76] and prostacyclin production, serum lipids, and BP using a mixture of alpha tocopherol and tocotrienols.[77]

Human studies of vitamin E in doses of 400 to 1,000 IU/day, although limited, have shown beneficial effects on improving insulin sensitivity,[78] lowering serum glucose,[8] inhibiting TxA_2,[70] increasing serum glutathione levels,[78] increasing intracellular magnesium,[78] improving arterial compliance (37–44%) (independent of arterial pressure),[81] reducing ED and vascular resistance,[81,82] and decreasing OxLDL.[82] However, reductions in BP in hypertensive subjects have been inconsistent, limited to small numbers of subjects, or it has been difficult to interpret the results for a variety of reasons.[78,79,83]

Barbagallo et al.[78] evaluated 24 hypertensive subjects in a double-blind, randomized, placebo-controlled study who received vitamin E 600 IU/day for 4 weeks. The BP in both treatment and placebo groups was decreased significantly (p<0.001 for SBP and p<0.005 for DBP), but both groups received furosemide 25 mg per day. The effects of vitamin E on BP cannot be interpreted in this study.

Palumbo et al.[79] administered 300 IU vitamin E per day to 142 treated hypertensive subjects in a randomized, open-labeled trial for 12 weeks. Clinic and 24-hour ABM showed no change in SBP and a small decrease in 24-hour ABM, DBP of −1.6 mm Hg (95% confidence intervals −2.8 to 0.4 mm Hg at p = 0.06). However, the mean BP at entry was 147/88 mm Hg in the vitamin E group, indicating reasonably good BP control by JNC-VI criteria. The day and night changes in mean ABM were not significant. The antihypertensive treatment clearly restricted the possibility of actually measuring a BP-lowering effect of vitamin E.

Iino et al.[83] performed a double-blind, placebo-controlled study of the effects of dl-alpha-tocopherol nicotinate in 94 hypertensive subjects with cerebral atherosclerosis. Subjects received 3,000 mg of the study vitamin for 4 to 6 weeks. In subjects with hypertension, the SBP declined from 151.0 +/− 22.1 mm Hg to 139.2 +/− 16.8 mm Hg ($p<0.05$), but DBP did not change.

If vitamin E has an antihypertensive effect, it is probably small and may be limited to untreated hypertensive patients or those with known vascular disease or other concomitant problems such as diabetes or hyperlipidemia.[81,82,83] However, vitamin E does improve ED through numerous mechanisms that could improve vascular health, reduce vascular and target organ damage that is BP-dependent or independent.[80,84] Hypertensive patients, compared to normotensive patients, have significantly lower plasma and cell content of vitamins E and C with increased lipid peroxidation.[84]

Notes

Chapter 1

1. "Why Should I Care?" American Heart Association http://www.americanheart.org/hbp/care.jsp. Viewed 7/19/02.
2. Chobanian, AV, et al. The Seventh Report of the Joint National Committee on Prevention, Detection, Evaluation, and Treatment of High Blood Pressure: The JNC 7 Report. *JAMA* 2003; 289(19): 2560–71.
3. Be careful when buying supplements. While there are many excellent brands that deliver exactly what they promise, there are others that do not. The key is to find independent certification that assures you're getting a high-quality product that contains everything it claims, is properly absorbed into your body, and is free of impurities, toxins, or side effects. Finding such certified products can be difficult without informed medical advice and supervision.

Chapter 2

1. The vascular endothelium has endocrine, paracrine, autocrine and intracrine functions.

Chapter 3

1. Addison W. *Can Med Assoc J*, 18:281–285, 1928. Cited in *Modern Nutrition in Health and Disease,* Vol. 2, 8th ed. Shils M, Olson J, Shike M, eds. Lea & Febiger, 1994, p. 1290.

2. *Modern Nutrition in Health and Disease*, vol. 2, 8th ed. Shils M, Olson J, Shike M eds. Lea & Febiger, 1994, p.1290.

3. *Modern Nutrition in Health and Disease*, vol. 2, 8th ed. Shils M, Olson J, Shike M eds. Lea & Febiger, 1994, p.1290.

4. Warner MG. Complementary and alternative therapies for hypertension. *Complementary Health Practice Review*. 2000;6:11–19.

5. Whelton PK, He J. Potassium in preventing and treating high blood pressure. *Semin Nephrol*. 1999;19:494–499.

6. Gu D, He J, Xigui W, Duan X, Whelton PK. Effect of potassium supplementation on blood pressure in Chinese: a randomized, placebo-controlled trial. *J Hypertens*. 2001;19:1325–1331. Barri YM, Wingo CS. The effects of potassium depletion and supplementation on blood pressure: a clinical review. *Am J Med Sci*. 1997;3:37–40.

7. Bucher HC, et al. Effects of dietary calcium supplementation on blood pressure. A meta-analysis of randomized controlled trials. *JAMA*. 1996;275:1016–1022. Griffith L, et al. The influence of dietary and nondietary calcium supplementation on blood pressure: an updated meta-analysis of randomized clinical trials. *Am J Hypertens*. 1999;12:84–92. Birkett NJ. Comments on a meta-analysis of the relation between dietary calcium intake and blood pressure. *Am J Epidemiol*. 1998;148:223–228.

8. Pfeifer M, et al. Effects of a short-term vitamin D(3) and calcium supplementation on blood pressure and parathyroid hormone levels in elderly women. *J Clin Endocrinol Metab*. 2001;86:1633–1637.

9. Weiss D. Cardiovascular disease: risk factors and fundamental nutrition. *Int J Integrative Med*. 2000;2:6–12.

10. Witteman JCM, et al. Reduction of blood pressure with oral magnesium supplementation in women with mild to moderate hypertension. *J Clin Nutr*. 1994;60:129–135.

11. Appel LJ. The role of diet in the prevention and treatment of hypertension. *Curr Atheroscler Rep*. 2000;2:521–528. Obarzanek E, et al. Dietary protein and blood pressure. *JAMA*. 1996;274:1598–1603. Stamler J, et al. Inverse relation of dietary protein markers. Findings for 10,020 men and women in the Intersalt study. Intersalt Cooperative Research Group. International study of salt and blood pressure. *Circulation*. 1996;94:1629–1634.

He J, Welton PK. Effect of dietary fiber and protein intake on blood pressure: a review of epidemiologic evidence. *Clin Exp Hypertens.* 1999;21: 785–796. Zhou B. The relationship of dietary animal protein and electrolytes to blood pressure. A study of three Chinese populations. *Int. J Epidemiol.* 1994;23:716–722.

12. Appel LJ. The role of diet in the prevention and treatment of hypertension. *Curr Atheroscler Rep.* 2000;2:521–528.

13. See, for example, Knapp HR, Fitzgerald GA. The antihypertensive effects of fish oil: a controlled study of polyunsaturated fatty acid supplements in essential hypertension. *New Engl J Med.* 1989;320:1037–1043: Bonaa KH, et al. Effect of eicosapentaenoic acid and docosahexaenoic acid on blood pressure in hypertension: a population based intervention trial from the Tromso study. *New Engl J Med.* 1990;322:795–801 and Toft I, et al. Effects of n-3 polyunsaturated fatty acids on glucose homeostasis and blood pressure in essential hypertension: a randomized, controlled trial. *Ann Intern Med.* 1995;123:911–918 Morris MC, et al. Does fish oil lower blood pressure? A meta-analysis of controlled trials. *Circulation.* 1993;88: 523–533.

14. Kromhout D, et al. The inverse relation between fish consumption and 20-year mortality from coronary heart disease. *N Engl J Med.* 1985;312: 1205–1209.

15. Knapp HR, Fitzgerald GA. The antihypertensive effects of fish oil: a controlled study of polyunsaturated fatty acid supplements in essential hypertension. *N Engl J Med.* 1989;320:1037–1043. *JANA* 28.

16. Mori TA, et al. Dietary fish as a major component of a weight-loss diet: effect on serum lipids, glucose and insulin metabolism in overweight hypertensive subjects. *Am J Clin Nutr.* 1999;70:817–825. *JANA* 28.

17. Weiss D. Cardiovascular disease; risk factors and fundamental nutrition. *Int J Integrative Med.* 2000;2:6–12. *JANA* 28.

18. Morris M, Sacks F, Rosner B. Does fish oil lower blood pressure? A meta-analysis of controlled trials. *Circulation.* 1993;88:523–533.

19. Bao DQ, et al. Effects of dietary fish and weight reduction on ambulatory blood pressure in overweight hypertensives. *Hypertension.* 1998;32: 710–717.

20. Ferrara LA, et al. Olive oil and reduced need for antihypertensive medications. *Arch Intern Med.* 2000;160:837–842. *JANA* 29.
21. Strazzullo P, et al. Changing the Mediterranean diet: effects on blood pressure. *J Hypertens.* 1986;4:407–412. *JANA* 29.
22. Ness AR, Chee D, Elliot P. Vitamin C and blood pressure—an overview. *J Hum Hypertens.* 1997;11:343–350.
23. Koh Et. Effect of vitamin C on blood parameters of hypertensive subjects. *J Okla State Med Assoc.* 1984;77:177–182.
24. Trout DL. Vitamin C and cardiovascular risk factors. *Am J Clin Nutr.* 1991;53:322–325. *JANA* 31.
25. Duffy SJ, et al. Treatment of hypertension with ascorbic acid. *Lancet.* 1999;354:2048–2049. *JANA* 31.
26. Fotherby MD, et al. Effect of vitamin C on ambulatory blood pressure and plasma lipids in older persons. *J Hypertens.* 2000;18:411–415. *JANA* 31.
27. Mongthuong T, et al. Role of coenzyme Q_{10} in chronic heart failure, angina, and hypertension. *Pharmacotherapy* 21(7):797–806, 2001.
28. Natural Medicines Comprehensive Database. 3rd ed. p. 303.
29. Langsjoen P, Willis R, Folkers K. Treatment of essential hypertension with coenzyme Q_{10}. *Mol Aspects Med.* 1994;15:S265–S272.
30. Asgary S, et al. Antihypertensive and anti-hyperlipidemic effects of Achillea wilelmsii. *Drug Exp Clin Res.* 2000;26:89–93. *JANA* 36.
31. Nijveldt RJ, et al. Flavonoids: a review of probable mechanisms of action and potential applications. *Am J Clin Nutr.* 2001;74:418–25.
32. Keniston R, Enriquez JI Sr. Relationship between blood pressure and plasma vitamin B_6 levels in healthy middle-aged adults. *Ann NY Acad Sci.* 1990;585:499–501.
33. Aybak M, et al. Effect of oral pyridoxine hydrochloride supplementation on arterial blood pressure in patients with essential hypertension. *Arzneimittelforschung.* 1995;45:1271–1273.
34. Singh RB, et al. Current zinc intake and risk of diabetes and coronary artery disease and factors associated with insulin resistance in rural and urban populations of North India. *J Am Coll Nutr.* 1998;17:564–570. *JANA* 25.

35. See, for example, DeBusk RM, Dietary supplements and cardiovascular disease. *Curr Atheroscler Rep.* 2000;2:508–514. Auer W, et al. Hypertension and hyperlipidaemia: garlic helps in mild cases. *Br J Clin Pract.* 1990;69:3–6. McMahon FG, Vargas R. Can garlic lower blood pressure? A pilot study. *Pharmacotherapy.* 1993;13:406–407. Lawson LD. Garlic: a review of its medical effects and indicated active compounds. In: Lawson LD, Bauer R, eds. *Phytomedicines of Europe: Chemistry and Biological Activity.* Washington, DC: American Chemical Society; 1998:176–209. Silagy CA, Neil AW. A meta-analysis of the effect of garlic on blood pressure. *J Hypertens.* 1994;12:463–468.

36. Ackerman RT, et al. Garlic shows promise for improving some cardiovascular risk factors. *Arch Intern Med.* 2001;161:813–824.

37. Suetsuna K, Nakano T. Identification of an antihypertensive peptide from peptic digest of wakame (Undaria pinnatifida). *J Nutr Biochem.* 2000;11:450–454.

38. Nakano T, et al. Hypotensive effects of wakame. *J Jpn Soc Clin Nutr.* 1998;20:92.

39. Krotkiewski M, et al. Effects of a sodium-potassium ion-exchanging seaweed preparation in mild hypertension. *Am J Hypertens.* 1991;4:483–488.

40. Pereira MA, Pins JJ. Dietary fiber and cardiovascular disease: experimental and epidemiologic advances. *Curr Atheroscler Rep.* 2000;2:494–502 Vuksan V, et al. Konjac-Mannan (Glucomannan) improves glycemia and other associated risk factors for coronary heart disease in type 2 diabetes. *Diabetes Care.* 1999;22:913–919. Kennan JM, et al. Oat ingestion reduces systolic and diastolic blood pressure among moderate hypertensives: a pilot trial. *J Fam Pract.* 2000. Pins JJ, et al. Whole grain cereals reduce antihypertensive medication need, blood lipid and plasma glucose levels. *J Am Coll Nutr.* 1999;18:529. Abstract.

41. Vuksan V, et al. Konjac-Mannan (Glucomannan) improves glycemia and other associated risk factors for coronary heart disease in type 2 diabetes. *Diabetes Care.* 1999;22:913–919. Kennan JM, et al. Oat ingestion reduces systolic and diastolic blood pressure among moderate hypertensives: a pilot trial. *J Fam Pract.* 2000.

42. Siani A, et al. Blood pressure and metabolic changes during dietary

L-arginine supplementation in humans. *Am J Hypertens.* 2000;13:547–551. Appel LJ, et al. A clinical trial of the effects of dietary patterns on blood pressure. *N Engl J Med.* 1997;336:1117–1124.

43. Siani A, et al. Blood pressure and metabolic changes during dietary L-arginine supplementation in humans. *Am J Hypertens.* 2000;13:547–551.

44. Fujita T, et al. Effects of increased adrenomedullary activity and taurine in young patients with borderline hypertension. *Circulation.* 1987;75: 525–532.

45. Paran E, Englehard YN. Effect of lycopene, an oral natural antioxidant, on blood pressure. *J Hypertens.* 2001;19:S74. Abstract P-1.204. Paran E, Englehard YN. Effect of tomato's lycopene on blood pressure, serum lipoproteins, plasma homocysteine and oxidative stress markers in grade I hypertensive patients. *Am J Hypertens.* 2001;14:141A. Abstract P-333.

46. Paran E, Englehard YN. Effect of tomato's lycopene on blood pressure, serum lipoproteins, plasma homocysteine and oxidative stress markers in grade I hypertensive patients. *Am J Hypertens.* 2001;14:141A. Abstract P-333.

47. Singh RB, et al. Can guava fruit intake decrease blood pressure and blood lipids? *J Hum Hypertens.* 1993;7:33–38.

Chapter 4

1. "How Can I Quit Smoking?" American Heart Association. http://216.185.122.5/presenter.jhtml?identifier=134. Viewed July 18, 2002.

Chapter 5

1. Appel LJ, Moore TJ, Obarzanek E, et al. A clinical trial of the effects of dietary patterns on blood pressure. *N Engl J Med.* 1997;336:1117–1124.

2. Resnick LM, et al. Factors affecting blood pressure responses to diet; the Vanguard Study. *Am J Hypertens.* 2000;13:956–965.

3. See for example: The Trials of Hypertension Prevention Collaborative

Research Group. The effects of nonpharmacologic interventions on blood pressure of persons with high normal levels. *JAMA.* 267:1213–1220. Sacks FM, Svetkey LP, Vollmer WM, Appel LJ, Bray GA, et al. Effects on blood pressure of reduced dietary sodium and the dietary approaches to stop hypertension (DASH) diet. *N Engl J Med.* 2001;344:3–10. McCarron DA, Oparil S, Chait A, et al. Nutritional management of cardiovascular risk factors: a randomized clinical trial. *Arch Intern Med.* 1997;157:169–177.

4. Appel LJ. The role of diet in the prevention and treatment of hypertension. *Curr Atheroscler Rep.* 2000;2:521–528. NHLBI. Clinical guidelines on the identification, evaluation, and treatment of overweight and obesity in adults—the evidence report. *J Obesity Res.* 1998;6:51S–209S. Reisen E, et al. Effect of weight loss without salt restriction of the reduction of blood pressure in overweight hypertensive patients. *N Engl J Med.* 1978;298:1–6. Conlin PR. Dietary modification and changes in blood pressure. *Curr Opin Nephrol Hypertens.* 2001;10:359–363. Tuck ML, et al. The effect of weight reduction on blood pressure, plasma rennin activity, and aldosterone levels in obese patients. *N Engl J Med.* 1981;304:930–933. McCarron DA, Reusser ME. Nonpharmalogic therapy in hypertension: from single components to overall dietary management. *Prog Cardiovasc Dis.* 1999;41:451–460.

5. Steven VJ, et al. Long-term weight loss and changes in blood pressure: results of the trials of hypertension prevention, phase II. *Ann Intern Med.* 2001;134:1–11.

6. Steven VJ, et al. Long-term weight loss and changes in blood pressure: results of the trials of hypertension prevention, phase II. *Ann Intern Med.* 2001;134:1–11.

7. McCarron DA, Reusser ME. Nonpharmalogic therapy in hypertension: from single components to overall dietary management. *Prog Cardiovasc Dis.* 1999;41:451–460.

8. Appel LJ. The role of diet in the prevention and treatment of hypertension. *Curr Atheroscler Rep.* 2000;2:521–528. Staessen J, et al. Body weight, sodium intake, and blood pressure. *J Hypertens.* 1989;7:S19–23.

Chapter 6

1. Ferrier LK et al. Alpha-linolenic acid and docosahexaenoic acid—enriched eggs from hens fed flaxseed: influence on blood lipids and platelet phospholipid fatty acids in humans. *Am J Clin Nutr.* 1995;62:81–86.

2. Hodgson JM, et al. Effects on blood pressure of drinking green and black tea. *J Hypertens.* 1999;17:457–463. Sung BH, et al. Prolonged increases in blood pressure by a single oral dose of caffeine in mildly hypertensive men. *Am J Hypertens.* 1994;7:755–758. Pincomb GA, et al. Acute blood pressure elevations with caffeine in men with borderline systemic hypertension. *Am J Cardiol.* 1996;77:270–274. Cavalcante JW, et al. Influence of caffeine on blood pressure and platelet aggregation. *Arq Bras Cardiol.* 2000;13:475–481.

3. Cavalcante JW, et al. Influence of caffeine on blood pressure and platelet aggregation. *Arq Bras Cardiol.* 2000;13:475–481.

4. The Sixth Report of the Joint National Committee on Prevention, Detection, Evaluation, and Treatment of High Blood Pressure. *Arch Intern Med.* 1997;157:24:2413–2446.

5. Fuchs FD, et al. Alcohol consumption and the incidence of hypertension: the atherosclerosis risk in communities study. *Hypertension.* 2001;37:1242–1250. World Hypertension League. Alcohol and hypertension: implications for management. *WHO Bull.* 1991;69:377–382. Altura BM, et al. Ethanol promotes rapid depletion of intracellular free Mg in cerebral vascular smooth muscle cells: possible relation to alcohol-induced behavioral and stroke-like effects. *Alcohol.* 1993;10:563–566. Zhang A, et al. Ethanol-induced contraction of cerebral arteries in diverse mammals and its mechanisms of action. *Eur J Pharmacol.* 1993;248:229–236.

6. The Sixth Report of the Joint National Committee on Prevention, Detection, Evaluation, and Treatment of High Blood Pressure. *Arch Intern Med.* 1997;157:24:2413–2446.

7. Fuchs FD, et al. Alcohol consumption and the incidence of hypertension: the atherosclerosis risk in communities study. *Hypertension.* 2001;37:1242–1250.

Chapter 7

1. US Department of Health and Human Services. *Physical Activity and Health: A Report of the Surgeon General.* Atlanta, GA: Centers for Disease Control and Prevention, National Center for Chronic Disease Prevention and Health Promotion; 1996.
2. American College of Sports Medicine. Physical activity, physical fitness and hypertension: position stand. *Med Sci Sports Exerc.* 1993;25:55–60.
3. Pescatello LS, Fargo AE, Leach CN, Scherzer HH. Short-term effect of dynamic exercise on arterial blood pressure. *Circulation.* 1991;83: 1557–1561.
4. Shephard RJ, Balady GJ. Exercise as cardiovascular therapy. *Circulation.* 99:963–972.
5. Shephard RJ, Balady GJ. Exercise as cardiovascular therapy. *Circulation.* 99:963–972.
6. Blair SN, Goodyear NN, Gibbons LW, Cooper KH. Physical fitness and incidence of hypertension in healthy normotensive men and women. *JAMA.* 1984;252:487–490.
7. Shephard RJ, Balady GJ. Exercise as cardiovascular therapy. *Circulation.* 99:963–972.
8. Sesso HD, Paffenbarger RS Jr., Lee IM. Physical activity and coronary heart disease in men. The Harvard Alumni Health Study. *Circulation.* 2000;102:975–980.

Chapter 8

1. Ghiadoni L, et al. Mental stress induces transient endothelial dysfunction in humans. *Circulation.* 11-14-2000:2473–2478.
2. Goldberg AD, et al. Ischemic, hemodynamic and neurohormonal responses to mental and exercise stress. *Circulation.* 1996;94:2402–2409.
3. Jonas BS. Are symptoms of anxiety and depression risk factors for hypertension? *Archives of Family Medicine.* 1997;6:43–49.
4. Cacioppo J. Biological costs of social stress in the elderly. Paper given at

a meeting of the American Psychological Association, Washington, DC, August 6, 2000.
5. Schneider RH, et al. A randomized controlled trial of stress reduction for hypertension in older African Americans. *Hypertension*. 1995;26:820.
6. King MS, Carr T, D'Cruz C. Transcendental meditation, hypertension and heart disease. *Aust Fam Physician*. 2002 Feb; 31(2):164–168.

Chapter 9

1. MacMahon S. Rodgers A. The effects of blood pressure reduction in older patients: an over-view of five randomized controlled trials in elderly hypertensives. *Clin Exp Hypertens*. 1993;15:967–978.
2. The Sixth Report of the Joint National Committee on Prevention, Detection, Evaluation, and Treatment of High Blood Pressure. *Arch Intern Med*. 1997;157;24:2413–2446.
3. The Seventh Report of the Joint National Committee on Prevention, Detection, Evaluation, and Treatment of High Blood Pressure. *J. Am. Med. Assoc.* 2003;289(19)2573–5.
4. The equivalent of 12.5 to 25 mg/day of hydrochlorothiazide or its equivalent.

Appendix

1. Warner MG. Complementary and alternative therapies for hypertension. *Complementary Health Practice Review*. 2000;6:11–19.
2. Ceriello A, Giugliano D, Quatraro A, et al. Antioxidants show an antihypertensive effect in diabetic and hypertensive subjects. *Clin Sci*. 1991;81:739–742.
3. Ness AR, Chee D, Elliot P. Vitamin C and blood pressure—an overview. *J Hum Hypertens*. 1997;11:343–350.
4. Solzbach U, Just H, Jeserich M, Hornig B. Vitamin C improves endothelial dysfunction of epicardial coronary arteries in hypertensive patients. *Circulation*. 1997;96:1513–1519.

5. Galley HF, Thornton J, Howdle PD, Walker BE, Webster NR. Combination oral antioxidant supplementation reduces blood pressure. *Clin Sci.* 1997;92:361–365.

6. Das UN. Minerals, trace elements, and vitamins interact with essential fatty acids and prostaglandins to prevent hypertension, thrombosis, hypercholesterolaemia and atherosclerosis and their attendant complications. *IRCS Med Sci.* 1985;13:684.

7. Weiss D. Cardiovascular disease: risk factors and fundamental nutrition. *Int J Integrative Med.* 2000;2:6–12.

8. Das UN, Horrobin DF, Begin ME, et al. Clinical significance of essential fatty acids. *Nutrition.* 1988;4:337.

9. Lal KJ, Dakshinamurti K. The relationship between low-calcium-induced increase in systolic blood pressure and vitamin B_6. *J Hypertens.* 1995;13:327–332.

10. DeBusk RM. Dietary supplements and cardiovascular disease. *Curr Atheroscler Rep.* 2000;2:508–514.

11. Auer W, Eiber A, Hertkorn E, Hoehfeld E, Koehrle U, Lorenz A, Mader F, Marx W, Otto G, Schmid-Otto B. Hypertension and hyperlipidaemia: garlic helps in mild cases. *Br J Clin Pract.* 1990;69:3–6.

12. McMahon FG, Vargas R. Can garlic lower blood pressure? A pilot study. *Pharmacotherapy.* 1993;13:406–407.

13. Lawson LD. Garlic: a review of its medical effects and indicated active compounds. In: Lawson LD, Bauer R, eds. *Phytomedicines of Europe: Chemistry and Biological Activity.* Washington, DC: American Chemical Society; 1998:176–209.

14. Pedraza-Chaverri J, Tapia E, Medina-Campos ON, de los Angeles Granados M, Franco M. Garlic prevents hypertension induced by chronic inhibition of nitric oxide synthesis. *Life Sci.* 1998;62:71–77.

15. Orekhov AN, Grunwald J. Effects of garlic on atherosclerosis. *Nutrition.* 1997;13:656–663.

16. Ernst E. Cardiovascular effects of garlic (Allium sativum): a review. *Pharmatherapeutica.* 1987;5:83–89.

17. Silagy CA, Neil AW. A meta-analysis of the effect of garlic on blood pressure. *J Hypertens.* 1994;12:463–468.

18. Silagy C, Neil A. Garlic as a lipid lowering agent: a meta-analysis. *J R Coll Physicians Lond.* 1994;28:39–45.

19. Ojewole JAO, Adewunmi CO. Possible mechanisms of antihypertensive effect of garlic: evidence from mammalian experimental models. *Am J Hypertens.* 2001;14:29A. Abstract.

20. Kleinjnen J, Knipschild P, Ter Riet G. Garlic, onions and cardiovascular risk factors: a review of the evidence from human experiments with emphasis on commercially available preparations. *Br J Clin Pharmacol.* 1989;28:535–544.

21. Reuter HD, Sendl A. Allium sativum and Allium ursinum: chemistry, pharmacology and medicinal applications. *Econ Med Plant Res.* 1994;6:55–113.

22. Mohamadi A, Jarrell ST, Shi SJ, Andrawis NS, Myers A, Clouatre D, Preuss HG. Effects of wild versus cultivated garlic on blood pressure and other parameters in hypertensive rats. *Heart Disease.* 2000;2:3–9.

23. Clouatre D. *European Wild Garlic: The Better Garlic.* San Francisco: Pax Publishing; 1995.

24. Sendl A, Elbl G, Steinke B, Redl K, Breu W, Wagner H. Comparative pharmacological investigations of Allium ursinum and Allium sativum. *Planta Med.* 1992;58:1–116.

25. Sendl A, Schliack M, Losu R, Stanislaus F, Wagner H. Inhibition of cholesterol synthesis in vitro by extracts and isolated compounds prepared from garlic and wild garlic. *Atherosclerosis.* 1992;94:79–85.

26. Wagner H, Elbl G, Lotter H, Guinea M. Evaluation of natural products as inhibitors of angiotensin I–converting enzyme (ACE). *Pharmacol Lett.* 1991;15–18.

27. Das I, Khan NS, Soornanna SSR. Potent activation of nitric oxide synthase by garlic: a basis for its therapeutic application. *Curr Med Res Opin.* 1994;13:257–263.

28. Torok B, Belagyi J, Rietz B, Jacob R. Effectiveness of garlic on the radical activity radical generating sytems. *Arzneimittelforschung.* 1994;44:608–611.

29. Jarrell ST, Bushehri N, Shi S-J, Andrawis N, Clouatre D, Preuss HG.

Effects of Wild Garlic (Allium ursinum) on blood pressure in SHR. *J Am Coll Nutr.* 1996;15:532. Abstract.

30. Mutsch-Eckner M, Meier B, Wright AD, Sticher O. Gammaglutamyl peptides from Allium sativum bulbs. *Phytochemistry.* 1992;31:2389–2391.

31. Meunier MT, Villie F, Jonadet M, Bastide J, Bastide P. Inhibition of angiotensin I–converting enzyme by flavonolic compounds: in vitro and in vivo studies. *Planta Med.* 1987;53:12–15.

32. Elkayam A, Mirelman D, Peleg E, Wilchck M, et al. The effects of allicin and enalapril in fructose-induced hyperinsulinemic, hyperlipidemic, hypertensive rats. *Am J Hypertens.* 2001;14:377–381

33. Ackermann RT, Mulrow CD, Ramirez G, Gardner CD, Morbidoni L, Lawrence VA. Garlic shows promise for improving some cardiovascular risk factors. *Arch Intern Med.* 2001;161:813–824.

34. Sherman DL, Keaney JF, Biegelsen ES, et al. Pharmacological concentrations of ascorbic acid are required for the beneficial effect on endothelial vasomotor function in hypertension. *Hypertension.* 2000;35:936–941.

35. Ting HH, Creager MA, Ganz P, Roddy MA, Haley EA, Timimi FK. Vitamin C improves endothelium-dependent vasodilation in forearm resistance vessels of humans with hypercholesterolemia. *Circulation.* 1997;95:2617–2622.

36. Taddei S, Virdis A, Ghiadoni L, Magagna A, Salvetti A. Vitamin C improves endothelium-dependent vasodilation by restoring nitric oxide activity in essential hypertension. *Circulation.* 1998;97:2222–2229.

37. Levine GN, Frei B, Koulouris SN, Gerhard MD, Keaney JF, Vita JA. Ascorbic acid reverses endothelial vasomotor dysfunction in patients with coronary artery disease. *Circulation.* 1996;93:1107–1113.

38. Heitzer T, Just H, Manzel T. Antioxidant vitamin C improves endothelial dysfunction in chronic smokers. *Circulation.* 1996;94:6–9.

39. Bates CJ, Walmsley CM, Prentice A, Finch S. Does vitamin C reduce blood pressure? Results of a large study of people aged 65 or older. *J Hypertens.* 1998;16:925–932.

40. Ness AR, Khaw K-T, Bingham S, Day NE. Vitamin C status and blood pressure. *J Hypertens.* 1996;14:503–508.

41. Moran JP, Cohen L, Green JM, Xu G, Feldman EB, Hames CG, Feld-

man DS. Plasma ascorbic acid concentrations relate inversely to blood pressure in human subjects. *Am J Clin Nutr.* 1993;57:213–217.

42. Duffy SJ, Gokce N, Holbrook M, et al. Treatment of hypertension with ascorbic acid. *Lancet.* 1999;354:2048–2049.

43. Schilling J, Holzer P, Guggenbach M, Gyurech D, Marathia K, Geroulanos S. Reduced endogenous nitric oxide in the exhaled air of smokers and hypertensives. *Eur Respir J.* 1994;7:467–471.

44. Emila H. Vitamin C and lowering of blood pressure: need for intervention trials? *J Hypertens.* 1991;9:1076–1077.

45. Feldman EB. The role of vitamin C and antioxidants in hypertension. *Nutrition and the M.D.* 1998;24:1–4.

46. Trout DL. Vitamin C and cardiovascular risk factors. *Am J Clin Nutr.* 1991;53:322–325.

47. Salonen JT, Salonen R, Ihanainen M, et al. Blood pressure, dietary fats, and antioxidants. *Am J Clin Nutr.* 1988;48:1226–1232.

48. Enster L, Dallner G. Biochemical, physiological and medical aspects of ubiquinone function. *Biochim Biophys Acta.* 1995;1271:195–204.

49. Simon JA. Vitamin C and cardiovascular disease: a review. *J Am Coll Nutr.* 1992;11:107–125.

50. Osilesi O, Trout DL, Ogunwole J. Glover EE. Blood pressure and plasma lipids during ascorbic acid supplementation in borderline hypertensive and normotensive adults. *Nutr Res.* 1991;11:405–412.

51. Lovat LB, Lu Y, Palmer AJ, Edwards R, Fletcher AE, Bulpitt CJ. Double blind trial of vitamin C in elderly hypertensives. *J Hum Hypertens.* 1993;7:403–405.

52. Ghosh SK, Ekpo EB, Shah IU, Girling AJ, Jenkins C, Sinclair AJ. A double-blind placebo controlled parallel trial of vitamin C treatment in elderly patients with hypertension. *Gerontology.* 1994;40:268–272.

53. Fotherby MD, Williams JC, Forster LA, Craner P, Ferns GA. Effect of vitamin C on ambulatory blood pressure and plasma lipids in older persons. *J Hypertens.* 2000;18:411–415.

54. Koh ET. Effect of vitamin C on blood parameters of hypertensive subjects. *J Okla State Med Assoc.* 1984;77:177–182.

55. Block G, Mangels AR, Patterson BH, Levander OA, Norkus E, Taylor

PR. Body weight and prior depletion affect plasma ascorbate levels attained on identical vitamin C intake: a controlled-diet study. *J Am Coll Nutr.* 1999;18:628–637.

56. Grossman M, Dobrev D, Himmel HM, Ravens U, Kirsh W. Ascorbic acid–induced modulation of venous tone in humans. *Hypertension.* 2001;37:949–954.

57. Yoshioka M, Aoyama K, Matsoshita T. Effects of ascorbic acid on blood pressure and ascorbic acid metabolism in spontaneously hypertensive rats. *Int J Vitam Nutr Res.* 1985;55:301–307.

58. Enstrom JE, Kanim LE, Klein M. Vitamin C intake and mortality among a sample of the United States population. *Epidemiology.* 1992;3:194–202.

59. Gale CR, Martyn CN, Winter PD, Cooper C. Vitamin C and risk of death from stroke and coronary heart disease in cohort of elderly people. *BMJ.* 1995;310:1563–1566.

60. Egan DA, Garg R, Wilt TJ, et al. Rationale and design of the arterial disease multiple intervention trial (ADMIT) pilot study. *Am J Cardiol.* 1999;83:569–575.

61. Block G, Mangels AR, Norkus EP, Patterson BH, Levander OA, Taylor PR. Ascorbic acid status and subsequent diastolic and systolic blood pressure. *Hypertension.* 2001;37:261–267.

62. Hajjar IM, George V, Kochar M. Effect of vitamin C supplementation on systolic, diastolic, pulse pressure and lipids: a randomized controlled trial. *Am J Hypertens.* 2001;14:143A. Abstract P-339.

63. Das UN. Hypertension and ascorbic acid. *Lancet.* 2000;355:1273.

64. Salonen R, Korpela H, Nyyssonen K, Porkkala E, Salonen JT. Reduction of blood pressure by antioxidant supplementation: a randomized double-blind clinical trial. *Life Chem Rep.* 1994;12:65–68.

65. Toivanan JL. Effects of selenium, vitamin E and vitamin C on human prostacyclin and thromboxane synthesis in vitro. *Prostaglandins Leukotrienes Med.* 1987;26:265–280.

66. Miller ER III, Appel LJ, Levander OA, Levine DM. The effect of antioxidant vitamin supplementation on traditional cardiovascular risk factors. *J Cardiovasc Risk.* 1997;4:19–24.

67. Cooke JP. Nutraceuticals for cardiovascular health. *Am J Cardiol.* 1998:82:43S–45S.

68. Hornig B, Arakawa N, Kohler C, Drexler H. Vitamin C improves endothelial function of conduit arteries in patients with chronic heart failure. *Circulation.* 1998;97:363–368.

69. Beetens JR, Herman AG. Ascorbic acid and prostaglandin formation. *Int J Vitam Nutr Res Suppl.* 1983;24:131–143.

70. Siow RC, Richards JP, Pedley KC, Leake DS, Mann GE. Vitamin C protects human vascular smooth muscle cells against apoptosis induced by moderately oxidized LDL containing high levels of lipid hydroperoxides. *Arterioscler Thromb Vasc Biol.* 1999;19:2387–2394.

71. Kendler BS. Nutritional strategies in cardiovascular disease control: an update on vitamins and conditionally essential nutrients. *Prog Cardiovasc Nurs.* 1999;14:124–129.

72. Newaz MA, Nawal NNA. Effect of ?-tocotrienol on blood pressure, lipid peroxidation and total antioxidant status in spontaneously hypertensive rats (SHR). *Clin Exp Hypertens.* 1999;21:1297–1313.

73. Newaz MA, Nawal NNA. Effect of a-tocopherol on lipid peroxidation and total antioxidant status in spontaneously hypertensive rats. *Am J Hypertens.* 1998;11:1480–1485.

74. Newaz MA, Nawal NNA, Muslim N, Gapor A. A-tocopherol increased nitric oxide synthase activity in blood vessels of spontaneously hypertensive rats. *Am J Hypertens.* 1999;12:839–844.

75. Igarashi T, Nakajima Y, Kobayashi M, Ohtake S. Anti-hypertensive action of DL-alpha-tocopheryl esters in rats. *Clin Sci Mol Med Suppl.* 1976;3:163s–164s.

76. Pezeshk A, Derick Dalhouse A. Vitamin E, membrane fluidity, and blood pressure in hypertensive and normotensive rats. *Life Sci.* 2000;67:1881–1889.

77. Koba K, Abe K, Ikeda I, Sugano M. Effects of alpha-tocopherol and tocotrienols on blood pressure and linoleic acid metabolism in the spontaneously hypertensive rat (SHR). *Biosci Biotechnol Biochem.* 1992;56:1420–1423.

78. Barbagallo M, Dominguez LJ, Tagliamonte MR, Resnick LM, Paolisso

G. Effects of vitamin E and glutathione on glucose metabolism. The role of magnesium. *Hypertension.* 1999;34:1002–1006.

79. Palumbo G, Avanzini F, Alli C, Roncaglioni C, et al. Effects of vitamin E on clinic and ambulatory blood pressure in treated hypertensive patients. *Am J Hypertens.* 2000;13:564–567.

80. Martin-Nrard F, Boullier A, Fruchart JC, Duriez P. Alpha tocopherol but not beta-tocopherol inhibits thrombin induced PKC activation and endothelin secretion in endothelial cells. *J Cardiovasc Risk.* 1998;5:339–345.

81. Mottram P, Shige H, Nestel P. Vitamin E improves arterial compliance in middle-aged men and women. *Atherosclerosis.* 1999;145:399–404.

82. Skyrme-Jones RA, O'Brien RC, Berry KL, Meredith IT. Vitamin E supplementation improves endothelial function in type I diabetes mellitus: a randomized, placebo-controlled study. *J Am Coll Cardiol.* 2000;36: 94–102.

83. Iino K, Abe K, Kariya S, Kimura H, Kusaba T, et al. A controlled, double-blind study of dl-alpha-tocopheryl nicotinate (Juvela-Nicotinate) for treatment of symptoms in hypertension and cerebral arteriosclerosis. *Jpn Heart J.* 1977;18:277–286.

84. Wen Y, Killalea S, McGettigan P, Freely J. Lipid peroxidation and antioxidant vitamins C and E in hypertensive patients. *IJMS.* 1996;165: 210–212.

85. Lal KJ, Dakshinamurti K. Calcium channels in vitamin B_6–deficiency-induced hypertension. *J Hypertens.* 1993;11:1357–1362.

86. Fregly MJ, Cade JR. Effect of pyridoxine and tryptophan, alone and in combination, on the development of deoxycorticosterone acetate–induced hypertension in rats. *Pharmacology.* 1995;50:298–306.

87. Lal KJ, Krishnamurti D, Thliverv J. The effect of vitamin B_6 on the systolic blood pressure of rats in various animal models of hypertension. *J Hypertens.* 1996;14:355–363.

88. Paulose CS, Dakshinamurti K, Packer S, Stephens NL. Hypertension in pyridoxine deficiency. *J Hypertens.* 1986;4:S174–S175.

89. Paulose CS, Dakshinamurti K, Packer S, Stephens NL. Sympathetic stimulation and hypertension in the pyridoxine-deficient adult rat. *Hypertension.* 1988;11:387–391.

90. Kleiger JA, Altshuler CH, Krakow G, Hollister C. Abnormal pyridoxine metabolism in toxemia of pregnancy. *Ann NY Acad Sci.* 1969;166: 288–296.

91. Brophy MH, Siiteri PK. Pyridoxal phosphate and hypertensive disorders of pregnancy. *Am J Obstet Gynecol.* 1975;121:1075–1079.

92. Brophy MH. Zinc, preeclampsia and g-aminobutyric acid. *Am J Obstet Gynecol.* 1990;163:242–243.

93. Brophy EM, Brophy MH. Pyridoxal phosphate normalization of the EEG in eclampsia. In: *Hypertension in Pregnancy.* Bologna; 1991:479.

94. Keniston R, Enriquez JI Sr. Relationship between blood pressure and plasma vitamin B_6 levels in healthy middle-aged adults. *Ann NY Acad Sci.* 1990;585:499–501.

95. Dakshinamurti K, Lal KJ. Vitamins and hypertension. *World Rev Nutr Diet.* 1992;69:40–73.

96. Aybak M, Sermet A, Ayyildiz MO, Karakilcik AZ. Effect of oral pyridoxine hydrochloride supplementation on arterial blood pressure in patients with essential hypertension. *Arzneimittelforschung.* 1995;45:1271–1273.

97. Bender DA. Non-nutritional uses of vitamin B_6. *Br J Nutr.* 1999;81:7–20.

98. Dakshinamurti K, Paulose CS, Viswanathan M. Vitamin B_6 and hypertension. *Ann NY Acad Sci.* 1990;575:241–249.

99. Dakshinamurti K, Lal KJ, Ganguly PK. Hypertension, calcium channel and pyridoxine (vitamin B_6). *Mol Cell Biochem.* 1998;188:137–148.

100. Lehninger AL. *Biochemistry: The Molecular Basis of Cell Structure and Function.* 2nd edition. New York: Worth; 1978:698.

101. Lal KJ, Dakshinamurti K, Thliveris J. The effect of vitamin B_6 on the systolic blood pressure of rats in various animal models of hypertension. *J Hypertens.* 1996;14:355–363.

102. Vasdev S., Ford CA, Parai S, Longerich L, Gadag V. Dietary vitamin B_6 supplementation attenuates hypertension in spontaneously hypertensive rats. *Mol Cell Biochem.* 1999;200:155–162.

103. Katz DL. *Nutrition in Clinical Practice.* Philadelphia: Lippincott Williams and Wilkins; 2001:370–371.

104. Paran E, Engelhard YN. Effect of lycopene, an oral natural antioxidant, on blood pressure. *J Hypertens.* 2001;19:S74. Abstract P-1.204.

105. Paran E, Engelhard YN. Effect of tomato's lycopene on blood pressure, serum lipoproteins, plasma homocysteine and oxidative stress markers in grade I hypertensive patients. *Am J Hypertens.* 2001;14:141A. Abstract P-333.

106. Digiesi V, Cantini F, Oradei A, Bisi G, Guarino GC, Brocchi A, Bellandi F, Mancini M, Littarru GP. Coenzyme Q_{10} in essential hypertension. *Mol Aspects Med.* 1994;15:S257–S263.

107. Langsjoen PH, Langsjoen AM. Overview of the use of CoQ_{10} in cardiovascular disease. *Biofactors.* 1999;9:273–284.

108. Singh RB, Niaz MA, Rastogi SS, Shukla PK, Thakur AS. Effect of hydrosoluble coenzyme Q_{10} on blood pressure and insulin resistance in hypertensive patients with coronary heart disease. *J Hum Hypertens.* 1999;13:203–208.

109. Digiesi V, Cantini F, Brodbeck B. Effect of coenzyme Q_{10} on essential hypertension. *Curr Ther Res.* 1990;47:841–845.

110. Morisco C, Trimarco B, Condorelli M. Effect of coenzyme Q_{10} therapy in patients with congestive heart failure: a long-term multicenter randomized trial. *Clin Investig.* 1993;71:S134–S136.

111. Kontush A, et al. Plasma ubiquinol is decreased in patients with hyperlipidemia. *Atherosclerosis.* 1997;129:119–126.

112. Yokoyama H, et al. Coenzyme Q_{10} protects coronary endothelial function from ischemia reperfusion injury via an antioxidant effect. *Surgery.* 1996;120:189–196.

113. Digiesi V, et al. Mechanism of action of coenzyme Q_{10} in essential hypertension. *Curr Ther Res.* 1992;51:668–672.

114. *Alternative Medicine Review.* 1996;Vol. I(3):171–174.

115. Yamagami T, Iwamoto Y, Folkers K, Blomqvist CG. Reduction by coenzyme Q_{10} of hypertension induced by deoxycorticosterone and saline in rats. *Int J Vitam Nutr Res.* 1974;44:487–496.

116. Garashi T, Nakajima Y, Tanaka M, Ohtake S. Effect of coenzyme Q_{10} on experimental hypertension in rats and dogs. *J Pharmacol Exp Ther.* 1974;189:149–156.

117. Iwamoto Y, Yamagami T, Folkers K, Blomqvist CG. Deficiency of coenzyme Q_{10} in hypertensive rats and reduction of deficiency by treatment with coenzyme Q_{10}. *Biochem Biophys Res Commun*. 1974;58:743–748.

118. Okamoto H, Kawaguchi H, Togashi H, Minami M, Saito H, et al. Effect of coenzyme Q_{10} on structural alterations in the renal membrane of stroke-prone spontaneously hypertensive rats. *Biochem Med Metabol Biol*. 1991;45:216–226.

119. Yamagami T, Takagi M, Akagami H, Kubo H, Toyama S, Okamoto T, Kishi T, Folkers K. Effect of coenzyme Q_{10} on essential hypertension, a double-blind controlled study. In: *Biomedical and Clinical Aspects of Coenzyme Q, Vol. 5*. Amsterdam: Elsevier; 1986:337–343.

120. Yamagami T, Shibata N, Folkers K. Study of coenzyme Q_{10} in essential hypertension. In: Folkers K, Yamamura Y, eds. *Biomedical and Clinical Aspects of Coenzyme Q, Vol. 1*. Amsterdam: Elsevier; 1977:231–242.

121. Tsuyusaki T, Noro C, Kikawada R. Mechanocardiography of ischemic or hypertensive heart failure. In: Yamamura Y, Folkers K, eds. *Biomedical and Clinical Aspects of Coenzyme Q, Vol. 2*. Amsterdam: Elsevier; 1980:273–288.

122. Richardson P, Drzewoski J, Ellis J, Shizukuishi S, Takemura K, Baker L, Folkers K. Reduction of elevated blood pressure by coenzyme Q_{10}. *Biomedical and Clinical Aspects of Coenzyme Q, Vol. 3*. Amsterdam: Elsevier; 1981:229–234.

123. Hamada M, Kazatani Y, Ochi T, Ito T, Kokubu T. Correlation between serum CoQ_{10} level and myocardial contractility in hypertensive patients. *Biomedical and Clinical Aspects of Coenzyme Q, Vol. 4*. Amsterdam: Elsevier; 1984:263–270.

124. Montaldo PL, Fadda G, Salis S, Satta G, Tronci M, DiCesare R, Reina R, Concu A. Effects of the prolonged administration of coenzyme Q_{10} in borderline hypertensive patients: a hemodynamic study. *Biomedical and Clinical Aspects of Coenzyme Q, Vol. 6*. Amsterdam: Elsevier; 1991:417–424.

125. Vasdev S, Ford CA, Parai S, et al. Dietary alpha-lipoic acid supple-

mentation lowers blood pressure in spontaneously hypertensive rats. *J Hypertens*. 2000;18:567–573.

126. Bierhaus A, Chevion S, Chevion M, Hoffman M, Quehenberger P, Illmer T, Luther T, Berentshtein E, Tritschler H, Muller M, Wahl P, Ziegler R, Nawroth PP. Advanced glycation end product–induced activation of Nf kappa B is suppressed by alpha lipoic acid in cultured endothelial cells. *Diabetes*. 1997;46:1481–1490.

127. Arivazhagan P, Juliet P, Panneerselvam C. Effect of dl alpha-lipoic acid on the status of lipid peroxidation and antioxidants in aged rats. *Pharmacol Res*. 2000;41:299–303.

128. Jacob S, Henriksen EJ, Schiemann AL, Simon I, Clancy DE, Tritschler HJ, et al. Enhancement of glucose disposal in patients with type 2 diabetes by alpha-lipoic acid. *Arzneimittelforschung*. 1995;45:872–874.

129. Henriksen EJ, Jacob S, Streeper RS, Fogt DL, Hokama JY, Tritschler HJ. Stimulation by a-lipoic acid of glucose transport activity in skeletal muscle of lean and obese zucker rats. *Life Sci*. 1997;61:805–812.

130. Busse E, Zimmer G, Schopohl B, Kornhuber B. Influence of a-lipoic acid on intracellular glutathione in vitro and in vivo. *Arzneimittelforschung*. 1992;42:829–831.

131. Phillips SA, Mirrlees D, Thornalley PJ. Modification of the glyoxalase system in streptozotocin-induced diabetic rats. *Pharmacology*. 1993;46:805–811.

132. Han D, Handelman G, Marcocci L, Sen CK, Roy S, Kobuchi H, et al. Lipoic acid increases de novo synthesis of cellular glutathione by improving cystine utilization. *Biofactors*. 1997;6:321–338.

133. Packer L. A-lipoic acid: a metabolic antioxidant which regulates NF-kB signal transduction and protects against oxidative injury. *Drug Metab Rev*. 1998;30:245–275.

134. Anero DR, Burghardt B. Cardiac membrane vitamin E and malondialdehyde levels in heart muscle of normotensive and spontaneously-hypertensive rats. *Lipids*. 1989;24:33–38.

135. Uysal M, Bulur H, Sener D, Oz H. Lipid peroxidation in patients with essential hypertension. *Int J Clin Pharmacol Ther Toxicol*. 1986;24:474–476.

136. Vodoevich UP. Effect of lipoic acid, biotin, and pyridoxine on blood content of saturated and unsaturated fatty acids in ischemic heart disease and hypertension. *Vopr Pitan.* 1983;5:14–16.

137. Hoffmann PC, Souchard JP, Nepveu F, Labidalle S. Thionitrites as potent donors of nitric oxide: example of S-nitroso-and S,S'-dinitrosodihydrolipoic acids. *C R Seances Soc Biol Fil.* 1996;190:641–650.

138. Kunt T, Forst T, Wilhelm A, Tritschler H, Pfuetzner A, Harzer O, Englebach M, Zschaebitz A, Stofft E, Beyer J. Alpha lipoic acid reduces expression of vascular cell adhesion molecule-1 and endothelial adhesion of human monocytes after stimulation with advanced glycation end products. *Clin Sci (Colch).* 1999;96:75–82.

139. Duke JA. *The Green Pharmacy: Herbs, Foods and Natural Formulas to Keep You Young. Anti-Aging Prescriptions.* Philadelphia: Rodale/St. Martin's Press; 2001:1–546.

140. Huxtable RJ. Physiologic actions of taurine. *Physiol Rev.* 1992;72: 101–163.

141. Ciehanowska B. Taurine as a regulator of fluid-electrolyte balance and arterial pressure. *Ann Acad Med Stetin.* 1997;43:129–142.

142. Fujita T, Ando K, Noda H, Ito Y, Sato Y. Effects of increased adrenomedullary activity and taurine in young patients with borderline hypertension. *Circulation.* 1987;75:525–532.

143. Birdsall TC. Therapeutic applications of taurine. *Altern Med Rev.* 1998;3:128–136.

144. Huxtable RJ, Sebring LA. Cardiovascular actions of taurine. *Prog Clin Biol Res.* 1983;125:5–37.

145. Harada H, Kitazaki K, Tsujino T, Watari Y, Iwata S, et al. Oral taurine supplementation prevents the development of ethanol-induced hypertension in rats. *Hypertens Res.* 2000;23:277–284.

146. Dawson R, Liu S, Jung B, Messina S, Eppler B. Effects of high salt diets and taurine on the development of hypertension in the stroke-prone spontaneously hypertensive rat. *Amino Acids.* 2000;19:643–665.

147. Fujita T, Sato Y. The antihypertensive effect of taurine in DOCA-salt rats. *J Hypertens Suppl.* 1984;2:S563–S565.

148. Fujita T, Sato Y. Changes in blood pressure and extracellular fluid with taurine in DOCA-salt rats. *Am J Physiol.* 1986;250:R1014–R1020.

149. Sato Y, Fujita T. Role of sympathetic nervous system in hypotensive action of taurine in DOCA-salt rats. *Hypertension.* 1987;9:81–87.

150. Fujita T, Sato Y. Hypotensive effect of taurine. Possible involvement of the sympathetic nervous system and endogenous opiates. *J Clin Invest.* 1988;82:993–997.

151. Trachtman H, Del Pizzo R, Rao P, Rujikarn N, Sturman JA. Taurine lowers blood pressure in the spontaneously hypertensive rat by a catecholamine independent mechanism. *Am J Hypertens.* 1989;2:909–912.

152. Petty MA, Kintz J, DiFrancesco GF. The effects of taurine on atherosclerosis development in cholesterol-fed rabbits. *Eur J Pharmacol.* 1990;180:119–127.

153. Sato Y, Ogata E, Fujita T. Hypotensive action of taurine in DOCA-salt rats—involvement of sympathaoadrenal inhibition and endogenous opiate. *Jpn Circ J.* 1991;55:500–508.

154. Ideishi M, Miura S, Sakai T, Sasaguri M, Misumi Y, Arakawa K. Taurine amplifies renal kallikrein and prevents salt-induced hypertension in DAHL rats. *J Hypertens.* 1994;12:653–661.

155. Nakagawa M, Takeda K, Yoshitomi T, Itoh H, Nakata T, Sasaki S. Antihypertensive effect of taurine on salt-induced hypertension. *Adv Exp Med Biol.* 1994;359:197–206.

156. Kohashi N, Okabayashi T, Hama J, Katori R. Decreased urinary taurine in essential hypertension. *Prog Clin Biol Res.* 1983;125:73–87.

157. Ando K, Fujita T. Etiological and physiopathological significance of taurine in hypertension. *Nippon Rinsho.* 1992;50:374–381.

158. Meldrum MJ, Tu R, Patterson T, Dawson R, Petty T. The effect of taurine on blood pressure and urinary sodium, potassium and calcium excretion. *Adv Exp Med Biol.* 1994;359:207–215.

159. Tanabe Y, Urata H, Kiyonaga A, Ikede M, Tanake H, Shindo M, Arakawa K. Changes in serum concentrations of taurine and other amino acids in clinical antihypertensive exercise therapy. *Clin Exp Hypertens.* 1989;11:149–165.

160. Gentile S, Bologna E, Terracina D, Angelico M. Taurine induced di-

uresis and natriuresis in cirrhotic patients with ascites. *Life Sci.* 1994;54: 1585–1593.

161. Mizushima S, Nara Y, Sawamura M, Yamori Y. Effects of oral taurine supplementation on lipids and sympathetic nerve tone. *Adv Exp Med Biol.* 1996;403:615–622.

162. Tao L, Rao MR. Effects of enalapril and taurine on left ventricular hypertrophy and arrhythmia in the renovascular hypertensive rat. *Yao Xue Xue Bao.* 1996;31:891–896.

163. Ji Y, Tao L, Rao MR. Effects of taurine and enalapril on blood pressure, platelet aggregation and the regression of left ventricular hypertrophy in two-kidney-one-clip renovascular hypertensive rats. *Yao Xue Xue Bao.* 1995;30:886–890.

164. Le OT, Elliott WJ. Mechanisms of the hypotensive effect of 3-N-butyl phthalide (BUPH): a component of celery oil. *Am J Hypertension.* 1992;40: 326A. Abstract.

165. Le OT, Elliot WJ. Dose response relationship of blood pressure and serum cholesterol to 3-N-butyl phthalide, a component of celery oil. *Clinical Research.* 1991;39:750A. Abstract.

166. Duke JA. *The Green Pharmacy Herbal Handbook.* Emmaus, Pennsylvania: Rodale; 2000:68–69.

167. Castleman M. *The Healing Herbs: The Ultimate Guide to the Curative Power of Nature's Medicines.* Emmaus, Pennsylvania: Rodale; 1991;105–107.

168. Heinerman J. *Heinerman's New Encyclopedia of Fruits and Vegetables.* Paramus, New Jersey: Prentice Hall; 1995:93–95.

169. Houston M. The Role of Vascular Biology, Nutrition and Nutraceuticals in the Prevention and Treatment of Hypertension. *JANA* 2002;Suppl 1:5–71.

170. Langsjoen P, Willis R, Folkers K. Treatment of essential hypertension with coenzyme Q_{10}. *Mol Aspects Med.* 1994;15:S265–S272.

171. Bousquet P, Feldman J, Bloch R, Schwartz T. Central cardiovascular effects of taurine: comparison with homotaurine and muscimol. *J Pharmacol Exp Ther.* 1981;219:213–218.

172. Suetsuna K, Nakano T. Identification of an antihypertensive peptide

from peptic digest of wakame (Undaria pinnatifida). *J Nutr Biochem.* 2000;11:450–454.

173. Nakazato T, Shikama T, Toma S, Nakajima Y, Masuda Y. Nocturnal variation in human sympathetic baroreflex sensitivity. *J Auton Nerv Syst.* 1998;70:32–37.

174. Dobson H, Muir M, Hume R. The effect of ascorbic acid on the seasonal variations in serum cholesterol levels. *Scott Med J.* 1984;29:176–182.

175. Bates CJ, Burr MK, St Ledger AS. Vitamin C high density lipoproteins and heart disease in elderly subjects. *Age Ageing.* 1979;8:177–182.

176. Siow RC, Richards JP, Pedley KC, Leake DS, Mann GE. Vitamin C protects human vascular smooth muscle cells against apoptosis induced by moderately oxidized LDL containing high levels of lipid hydroperoxides. *Arterioscler Thromb Vasc Biol.* 1999;19:2387–2394.

Index

Achillea wilhelmsii, 74
adrenaline (epinephrine), 177, 180
aerobic exercise, 159–62, 169
African-Americans, 40–41, 182, 208
aging, 19, 40
alcohol, 11, 41, 96, 152–54, 179, 222
aldosterone, 38, 206
allicin, 78–79, 220
alpha-beta blockers, 204–205
alpha$_1$ blockers, 203–204
alpha linolenic acid (ALA), 60, 61, 62, 63, 225–29
alpha lipoic acid, 83–84
Alzheimer's disease, 37
American Heart Association, 7, 11, 97, 99
American Journal of Clinical Nutrition, 62
American Nutraceutical Association, 93
American Society of Hypertension, 221
angina, 36, 69
angiotensin-converting enzyme (ACE), 38, 47
angiotensin-converting enzyme inhibitors (ACE inhibitors) (ACEIs), 47, 205–207
natural, 57, 78–79, 81–82, 87
angiotensin I, 38, 205
angiotensin II, 38, 205–206, 210
angiotensin II receptor blockers (ARBs), 47, 210–11
animal protein, 57–58, 132, 139
antihypertensive medications, ix, x, 11, 99, 186–218, 219, 222
  alpha-beta blockers, 204–205
  alpha blockers, 191, 203–204
  angiotensin-coverting enzyme inhibitors (ACE inhibitors) (ACEIs), 47, 205–207
  angiotensin II receptor blockers (ARBs), 47, 210–11
  beta blockers, 47, 191, 199–202
  calcium channel blockers, 47, 191, 207–10
  central alpha agonists, 47, 191, 197–99
  chemical, generic, and trade names, 192
  consulting your physician about, 105

279

antihypertensive medications (*cont.*)
  cost of, 8
  diuretics, 47, 191, 193–97
  effectiveness of, 186–87
  guidelines for prescribing, 187–89
  one-drug or combined drug approaches, 191, 220
  postganglionic neuron inhibitors, 212
  questions to ask your physician before taking, 213–14
  side effects of, 8, 187, 194–214
  types of, 189–91
  vasodilators, 47, 202–203
antioxidants, 10, 18, 46, 68, 72, 74, 83, 84
  see also vitamin E; *specific antioxidants, e.g.* vitamin C
anxiety, 181–82
aorta, 14
  aneurysm, 34
apigenin, 78
Archives of Internal Medicine, 64–65
arteries, 3, 16–17
  endothelium, *see* endothelium
  hardening of (atherosclerosis), 4, 20–21, 26, 27, 34, 73, 119, 208
  the media, 16, 17
  narrowed (vasoconstriction), 20–21, 24, 27
arterioles, 19, 26, 39
arteriosclerosis, 20
atherosclerosis (hardening of the arteries), 4, 20–21, 26, 27, 34, 73, 119, 208
Atherosclerosis Risk in Communities study, 153
ATP (adenosine triphosphate), 55
AV nicking, 39

baking powder (sodium aluminum sulfate), 110

baking soda (sodium bicarbonate), 110
Benson, Dr. Herbert, 182
beta blockers, 47, 191, 199–202
  natural, 88
beta-carotene, 68
biotin, 84
blood clots, 21, 27–28, 74, 158
blood clotting, 18, 73
blood pressure, 21–28
  defined, 21
  diastolic (DBP), 5, 21–24, 27–28
  hypertension, *see* hypertension
  method for checking, 4–5, 6, 43, 90–92
  normal, 6
  prehypertension, 6
  systolic (SBP), 5, 21–26
blood vessels, 34
  hypertension as disease of the, 30
  see also specific vessels, e.g. arteries; capillaries
blood viscosity, 23, 177
blood volume, 21
body mass index (BMI), 116–17
brain, hypertension's effects on the, 36–37
breakfast, 121, 124
brine, 110

caffeine, 11, 42, 96–97, 150–52, 222
calcium, x, 51–53, 132, 137–38
  food sources of, 53, 138
  other minerals and, 56–57, 136
calcium channel blockers (CCBs), 47, 191, 207–10
  natural, 83, 87
cancer, 2, 97
canola oil, 142, 144
capillaries, 3, 18
carbohydrates, 132, 139, 144–46
  complex, 132, 145–46

Index

refined, 42
simple, 145
cardiac output (CO), 21
cardiomegaly, 35
cardiovascular system, 3, 14–19
  benefits of exercise for, 157–58
catechins, 74
catecholamines, 212
celery, 77–78, 132, 149, 230
central alpha antagonists, 47, 191, 197–99
  natural, 86
central postsynaptic alpha$_2$ receptor, 197
Chicken Waldorf Salad Sandwich, 126
cholesterol, serum, 19, 37, 69, 73, 146, 157
  HDL ("good), 35, 76, 77, 80, 143, 147, 157
  LDL ("bad"), 35, 69, 73, 74, 80, 143, 147, 157
  VLDL (very low density lipoprotein), 35, 53
cigarette smoking, *see* smoking
Circulation, 62
coenzyme Q$_{10}$, x, 10, 45, 69–71, 220, 230–36
complementary and integrative medicine, 9
congestive heart failure, 2, 32, 69, 186
coronary artery disease, 35–36, 76
coronary heart disease, 2, 97, 186
  exercise to protect against, 166–67
corticosteroids, 133
cortisol, 153, 177

daidzein, 74
DASH (Dietary Approaches to Stop Hypertension) diets, 10, 12, 100–130, 154, 221
  basic guidelines, 121–22
  benefits of, 92
  DASH-I, 10–11, 92, 101–103, 221
  DASH-II, 11, 92, 103–104, 108–109, 221
  getting started, 123
  overview, 105–107
  recipes, 123–30
  sample menus, 121–22
  1,600 calorie, 120
  tips for incorporating fruits and vegetables, 107–108
  VasoGuard Therapy combined with, 154
dementia, 37
depression, 181–82
designing your own antihypertensive diet, 131–54
  guidelines for, 131–33
  reminder about not duplicating VasoGuard Therapy *and* supplements, 154
diabetes, 19, 37, 179
  Type I, 118
  Type II, 76
diastolic blood pressure, 5, 21–24, 27–28
diets, ix
  crash, 119
  DASH (Dietary Approaches to Stop Hypertension) diets, *see* DASH (Dietary Approaches to Stop Hypertension) diets
  designing your own, *see* designing your own antihypertensive diet
dinner, 122
diuretics, 47, 191, 193–97
  natural, 86, 134
docosahexaenoic acid (DHA), 60, 63, 140
double-blind, randomized studies, 64–65
drugs, recreational, 41–42

eclampsia, 26, 29
Eggs with Spinach and Fresh Salsa, Scrambled, 124–25
eicosapentaenoic acid (EPA), 60, 63, 140
elderly, antihypertensive medications and the, 186, 208
embolus, 21
endothelium, 16, 17–18, 19, 72, 157–58
   dysfunction, 4, 19–20, 24, 27, 28, 34, 67, 80, 83, 97, 178
entrée recipes, 126–29
epinephrine (adrenaline), 177, 180
essential hypertension, 5, 30
exercise, ix, 42, 94, 155–76, 222
   aerobic, 159–62, 169
   benefits for cardiovascular system, 157–58
   calorie expenditure chart, 167
   caution, 173
   combining aerobic and resistance, 160–61, 169
   duration of, 166–68
   effect on blood pressure, 156, 157
   frequency, 161–63
   intensity, 163–66
   making the commitment to, 169
   resistance, 160–61, 162, 165–66, 169
   for stress management, 158, 185
   tips for successful exercise program, 173–75
   Ultimate Exercise Prescription, 170–73

fats, serum level of, 76
fatty acids (dietary fats), 10, 42, 45, 57, 58–60, 132, 139, 140–44
   omega-3, *see* omega-3 polyunsaturated fatty acids
   omega-6, *see* omega-6 fatty acids
   omega-9, 140, 142
   see also specific types of fatty acids
fiber, 80, 146–48
fibrosis, 24, 27, 34
fight-or-flight response, 177–78
fish and fish oils:
   as source of omega-3 fatty acids, 58, 61, 62, 141–42
   see also omega-3 polyunsaturated fatty acids
flavonoids, 10, 73–75, 82
flaxseeds and flaxseed oil, 64, 140, 142
free radicals, *see* antioxidants
Fruit Medley Smoothie, 129–30

gamma linolenic acid (GLA), 64
garlic, 78–79, 132, 148, 220, 236–38
gender, 41
genetics, 19, 30, 40
genistein, 74
glossary, 214–18
glucose, blood, 69, 118, 145, 157
green tea, 74
guava fruit, 84–85, 132, 149

Harvard Alumni Health Study, 166
hawthorn berry, 81–82
Health Nut Toast, 125
heart, 3, 15
   damage from hypertension to the, 35–36
heart attack, ix, 2, 4, 7, 26, 28, 32, 36, 179, 186
heart disease, coronary, 2, 97, 186
   exercise to protect against, 166–67
heart rate, 177, 199
   target, 163–65
herbs, 84
high blood pressure, *see* hypertension
homocysteine levels in the blood, 37

Index

hormonal factors affecting blood pressure, 26, 28
Houston, Dr. Mark, experience in standard medicine, 9
hydrogenated fats, 143
hypertension:
  defined, 5
  as disease of the blood vessels, 30
  essential, 5, 30
  harm caused by excess pressure, 3–4, 19–21, 33–39
  Hypertension Institute Program, see Hypertension Institute Program
  life expectancy and, 36
  medications, *see* antihypertensive medications
  research on, *see* research on hypertension
  risk factors, 40–43, 187–88
  secondary, 5, 30–31, 43
  signs of, 43–44
  stages of, blood pressure measurements and, 7
  treatment of, *see specific components of treatment, e.g.* antihypertensive medications; exercise; VasoGuard Therapy
  white coat, 32–33
  see also blood pressure
Hypertension, 62
Hypertension Institute, 9
Hypertension Institute Program, 8–9, 89–99
  components of, 11, 12–13, 89–99, 221
  research behind, 11–12, 221
hypertrophy of artery wall, 23

insulin, 118–19, 145
insulin receptor site, 118
insulin resistance, 76, 118–19
insulin sensitivity, 61, 69, 80
International, European, and American Societies of Hypertension, 11
International Journal for Vitamin and Nutrition Research, 69
Intersalt Study, 57

Joint National Committee on Prevention, Detection, Evaluation, and Treatment of High Blood Pressure, 6, 11, 99, 187, 191, 221
Journal of Human Hypertension, 84
Journal of Hypertension, 67

kidney disease, 37–39, 186, 208
kidney failure, ix, 2, 4, 32
Korotkoff sounds, 6

L-arginine, 81
L-carnitine, 82–83
left-ventricular hypertrophy, 35, 208
loneliness, 182
lumen, 23
lunch, 122
lycopene, 84, 133, 149, 238

magnesium, x, 45, 54–56, 79, 132, 136–37, 220
  food sources of, 56, 136–37
  other minerals and, 56–57, 136
Mahesh, Maharishi, 183
maitake mushrooms, 132, 148
medications:
  affecting blood pressure, 41–42
  antihypertensive, *see* antihypertensive medications
  chemical, generic, and trade names, 192

medications (*cont.*)
  high-sodium, 112
  questions to ask your physician before taking, 213–14
Mediterranean Veal Stew, 127–28
minerals, 10
  see also specific minerals
mitochondria, 69
monounsaturated fatty acids (MUFAs), 59, 64, 65, 132, 140, 142, 144
MSG (monosodium glutamate), 110
mushrooms, 132, 148
myocardial infarction, *see* heart attack

n-acetyl cysteine, 83
National Health and Nutrition Examination Survey, 66, 181
National Heart, Lung and Blood Institute, 101–102
natriuresis, 57
New England Journal of Medicine, 60, 61
nitric oxide, 18, 65, 83
norepinephrine, 177
nutraceuticals, x, 10, 46, 47–88
  defined, 9
nutrition, *see* diets; *specific nutrients and supplements*

obesity, *see* weight, overweight and obesity
oleic acid, 64
olive oil, x, 64–65, 140, 142, 144
omega-3 polyunsaturated fatty acids, x, 57, 58–63, 132, 140–42
  benefits of, 61, 140–41
  food sources of, 59, 63, 141–42
  types of, 60
omega-6 fatty acids, 57, 59, 60, 64, 140, 142–43

omega-9 fatty acids, 140, 142
overeating in response to stress, 179
oxidative stress, 18, 69

Pauling, Dr. Linus, 65
peripheral artery disease, 26
physician:
  consulting your, 48, 105, 159, 173, 176, 221
  "doctor talk" definitions, 214–18
  guidelines for prescribing antihypertensive medications for, 187–89
  questions to ask, before taking any medication, 213–14
  regular doctor visits, 89–92
plaque, arterial, 20, 23, 24, 27, 28
platelets, 18, 177
polyunsaturated fatty acids (PUFAs), 59, 64, 132, 143
postganglionic neuron inhibitors, 212
potassium, x, 48–50, 132, 133–35, 153
  food sources of, 50, 135
  other minerals and, 49, 56–57, 132, 136
  sodium and, 49, 56–57, 132
preeclampsia (toxemia), 26, 29
pregnancy, 26, 28–29
processed foods, 114, 145
progressive relaxation, 182–83
prostaglandin E_1, 54–55
protein, 57–58, 139–40
psychological factors affecting blood pressure, 25, 28
pyridoxine (vitamin B_6), 75–76, 240–43

quercetin, 74

race, 40–41

African-Americans and hypertension, 40–41, 182, 191, 208
recipes, 123–30
red wine, 74
relaxation response, 182–83
renin-angiotensin-aldosterone system, 38, 76, 205, 206, 210
research on hypertension, x, 9–10, 45, 220, 224–52
  see also specific subject matter of hypertension research
resistance exercise, 160–61, 162, 165–66, 169
risk factors for hypertension, 40–43, 187–88

Salmon, Tropical Roasted, 128–29
Salsa, Scrambled Eggs with Spinach and Fresh, 124–25
salt, 109–10
  see also sodium
saturated fatty acids, 42, 45, 57, 59, 60, 132, 140, 143–44
Scrambled Eggs with Spinach and Fresh Salsa, 124–25
seaweed, wakame, 79–80, 132, 149, 220
secondary hypertension, 5, 30–31, 43
  accelerated and malignant, 32
selenium, 68
shiitake mushrooms, 132, 148
silent killer, hypertension as, ix, 1–2
Smoked Turkey Wrap with Avocado, 126–27
smoking, 11, 25–26, 28, 42, 97–99, 179, 222
Smoothie recipes, 129–30
snacks, 122
sodium, 26, 42, 45, 119, 132, 153
  DASH-II, restriction as part of, 103–104, 108–109, 221
  other minerals and, 49, 56–57, 132, 136
  potassium and, 49, 56–57, 132
  restriction, 11, 103–104, 108–16
soy, 74
sphygmomanometer, 4–5
spices, 115–16
Spinach and Fresh Salsa, Scrambled Eggs with, 124–25
statistics on Americans with hypertension, ix, 2–3, 7–8, 219, 222–23
stress, 11, 25, 26, 28, 43
  anxiety and, 181–82
  body's response to, 177–78
  chronic, 179
  depression and, 181–82
  de-stressing your life, 95–96, 177–85, 222
  exercise to manage, 158, 185
  harmful effects of, 177, 178–79
  loneliness and, 182
  mental compared to physical, 179–80
  other methods of relieving, 185
  symptoms of, 180–81
stroke, ix, 2, 4, 7, 28, 32, 36–37, 97, 186
sunflower oil, 64–65
supplements:
  guidelines for designing your own antihypertensive diet, 133
  VasoGuard Therapy, *see* VasoGuard Therapy
  see also specific supplements
sympathetic nervous system, 177, 178
systemic vascular resistance (SVR), 21
systolic blood pressure, 5, 21–26

target heart rate, 163–65

taurine, 82, 239–40
thrombus, 21
Toast, Health Nut, 125
tobacco products, 11, 25–26, 28, 42, 97–99, 179, 222
tocopherols, 72
tocotrienols, 72
Tofu Fruit Smoothie, 130
toxemia, 26, 29
Transcendental Meditation, 183–85
trans fatty acids, 42, 45, 132, 143–44
treatment of hypertension, *see specific components of treatment, e.g.* antihypertensive medications; exercise; *Hypertension Institute Program;* VasoGuard Therapy
triglycerides, 35, 147, 157
Tropical Fruit Smoothie, 129
Tropical Roasted Salmon, 128–29
Turkey Wrap with Avocado, Smoked, 126–27
type A personalities, 25

unsaturated fatty acids, 59, 60
uremia, 38

Vanguard Study, 104–105
vascular dementia, 37
vascular disease, 20
  see also stroke; *specific forms, e.g.* atherosclerosis
vasoconstriction of the arteries, 20–21, 24, 27
vasodilators, 47, 202–203
  natural, 86–87
VasoGuard Therapy, 92–94, 154, 220, 221
  combining with DASH diet, 154
Vaso-Guard Therapy, 10
Veal Stew, Mediterranean, 127–28
vegetable protein, 57–58, 139–40
veins, 3
venules, 19
vision problems, ix, 4, 39
vitamin B_6 (pyridoxine), 75–76, 240–43
vitamin C, x, 10, 45, 65–68, 220, 243–50
  food sources of, 68
vitamin D, 53–54
vitamin E, 68, 71–73, 250–52
vitamin K, 73
vitamins, 10, 46
  see also specific vitamins

wakame seaweed, 79–80, 132, 149, 220
water, 148, 175
water pills (diuretics), 47, 191, 193–97
weight:
  apple obesity, 30
  benefits of weight loss, 116–19
  body mass index (BMI), 116–17
  exercise and weight control, 158
  ideal, ix, 94–95, 222
  loss, 11, 116–20, 221, 222
  overweight and obesity, 24–25, 42, 94–95
white coat hypertension, 32–33
whole foods, 46
World Health Organization, 11, 99, 221

zinc, 76–77, 132, 138–39

ABOUT THE AUTHORS

Mark Houston, M.D., SCH, ABAAM, FACP, FAHA graduated *phi beta kappa* and *summa cum laude* from Rhodes College in Memphis, Tennessee, with a BA in chemistry and was a semifinalist as a Rhodes Scholar. He graduated with highest honors and the Alpha Omega Alpha honorary society distinction from Vanderbilt Medical School. He completed his medical internship and residency at the University of California, San Francisco, and then returned to Vanderbilt Medical Center where he was chief resident in medicine and received the Hillman Award for Best Teacher. Dr. Houston specializes in hypertension, lipid disorders, prevention and treatment of cardiovascular diseases, nutrition, clinical age management, and general internal medicine with an active clinical and research practice. He is presently associate clinical professor of medicine, Vanderbilt University School of Medicine, and director of the Hypertension Institute, Vascular Biology and the Life Extension Institute, Saint Thomas Medical Group, Saint Thomas Hospital and Health Services, in Nashville, Tennessee. He is staff physician of the Vascular Institute of Saint Thomas Hospital.

Dr. Houston is board certified by the American Board of Internal Medicine, the American Society of Hypertension as a specialist in clinical hypertension (SCH), and the American Board of Anti-Aging Medicine (ABAAM). He will also receive a masters of science degree in clinical nutrition from the University of Bridgeport, Connecticut, in 2003. He is a Fellow in the American College of Physicians (FACP), Fellow of the National Council on High Blood Pressure, and Fellow of the American Heart Association (FAHA). He is on the editorial board and is chair of the Medical Advisory Board of the American Nutraceutical Association (ANA) and editor-in-chief for the *Journal of the American*

Nutraceutical Association (JANA). He is on the board of trust and executive board for the Consortium of Southeastern Hypertension Control (COSEHC). He has published over 130 medical articles and monographs in peer-reviewed journals. Dr. Houston has authored two bestselling handbooks, *Handbook of Antihypertensive Therapy* and *Vascular Biology for the Clinician*.

Barry Fox, Ph.D., and Nadine Taylor, M.S., R.D., are a husband-and-wife writing team with more than thirty books to their credit. Their works include *The Arthritis Cure*, a *New York Times* #1 bestselling blockbuster that has sold over 1 million copies. They've also written over 160 articles for various magazines.

Barry is currently a professor in the Anti-Aging Concentration at the University of Integrated Studies and chair of the American Nutraceutical Association's Consumer Affairs Council. Nadine, a registered dietitian, is chair of the American Nutraceutical Association's Women's Health Council.

Among the books Barry and Nadine have authored or coauthored are *The Arthritis Cure* (St. Martin's, 1997), *Managing Menopause Without Drugs* (Penguin, 2003), *25 Natural Ways to Relieve PMS* (Contemporary Books, 2002), *What Your Doctor May Not Tell You About Migraines* (Warner Books, 2001), *Syndrome X* (Simon & Schuster, 2000), *Arthritis for Dummies* (IDG Books, 2000), *The 20/30 Fat and Fiber Diet Plan* (HarperCollins, 1999), *Cancer Talk* (Broadway Books, 1999), and *Diana and Dodi: A Love Story* (Tallfellow, 1998). Their books and articles—covering various aspects of physical and mental health, as well as business, biography, law, and other topics—have been translated into twenty languages.

You can learn more about Barry and Nadine at their Web site: www.Taylor-Fox.com.

ALSO AVAILABLE FROM WARNER BOOKS

OTHER TITLES FROM THE BESTSELLING SERIES WHAT YOUR DOCTOR MAY NOT TELL YOU ABOUT™...

AUTOIMMUNE DISORDERS
The Revolutionary Drug-free Treatments for Thyroid Disease • Lupus • MS • IBD • Chronic Fatigue • Rheumatoid Arthritis, and Other Diseases

BREAST CANCER
How Hormone Balance Can Help Save Your Life

CHILDREN'S VACCINATIONS
Learn What You Should—and Should Not—Do to Protect Your Kids

CIRCUMCISION
Untold Facts on America's Most Widely Performed—and Most Unnecessary—Surgery

FIBROIDS
New Techniques and Therapies—Including Breakthrough Alternatives

FIBROMYALGIA
The Revolutionary Treatment That Can Reverse the Disease

HPV AND ABNORMAL PAP SMEARS
Get the Facts on This Dangerous Virus—Protect Your Health and Your Life!

more...

KNEE PAIN AND SURGERY
Learn the Truth About MRIs and Common Misdiagnoses—
and Avoid Unnecessary Surgery

MENOPAUSE
The Breakthrough Book on Natural Hormone Balance

MIGRAINES
The Breakthrough Program That Can Help End Your Pain

OSTEOPOROSIS
Help Prevent—and Even Reverse—the Disease
That Burdens Millions of Women

PARKINSON'S DISEASE
A Holistic Program for Optimal Wellness

PEDIATRIC FIBROMYALGIA
A Safe, New Treatment Plan for Children

PREMENOPAUSE
Balance Your Hormones and Your Life from Thirty to Fifty